50 things you can do today to manage insomnia

Wendy Green

Foreword by Dr Chris Idzikowski,

Director of the Edinburgh Sleep Centre

PERSONAL HEALTH GUIDES

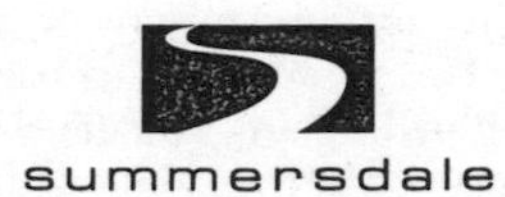

50 THINGS YOU CAN DO TODAY TO MANAGE INSOMNIA

Summersdale Publishers Ltd
46 West Street
Chichester
West Sussex
PO19 1RP
UK

www.summersdale.com

Printed and bound in Great Britain

ISBN: 978-1-84024-723-7

To my husband Gordon, for being so supportive

Acknowledgements

I'd like to thank Dr Chris Idzikowski, director of the Edinburgh Sleep Centre, for his expert help. I'd also like to thank Dr Neil Stanley of Norfolk and Norwich University Hospital for giving his expert opinion on various topics.

I'm also grateful to Jennifer Barclay and Lucy York at Summersdale for being so supportive and easy to work with during the writing of this book. Finally, I'd like to thank Laura Booth, the freelance editor who helped me to improve the overall organisation of the book.

Contents

Author's Note

For most of my life I've taken sleep for granted. Apart from the occasional sleepless night, usually when sleeping in unfamiliar surroundings, I was a sound sleeper. But a couple of years ago, as my life became increasingly busy, I began to suffer from sleepless nights more often. No doubt going through the menopause and having night sweats played a part, but I suddenly found that going to bed and sleeping right through until morning became a rarity rather than the norm. I now know from experience that there's nothing more frustrating than going to bed and lying awake, tossing and turning for hours on end, unable to switch off. Then, even if you finally manage to fall asleep, there are times when you find yourself awake again in the early hours, plagued by thoughts and worries that refuse to go away.

Whilst doing the research for this book, I realised that I experience most of my sleep problems when I haven't allowed myself to wind down at night; often it's because I've worked on the computer during the evening, and my mind has gone into 'overdrive'. I've also realised that sometimes I wasn't taking time during the day to think through any issues or worries, so they would resurface during the early hours, demanding my attention, when all I wanted to do was sleep!

Nowadays I try to relax for at least two hours before going to bed. If I have any concerns I try to sort them out in my head before I turn in. On the nights when I still have trouble switching off, I find a sprinkling of lavender oil on my pillow really helps me to relax. In the course of writing this book, I've learned that most sleep problems are due to some aspect of daily life being out of balance – for example through overwork, lack of exercise or too much caffeine. Of course there are other causes, including the use of certain medications, some medical conditions, mental health problems and sleep disorders. But generally, what we do during our waking hours affects the quality of our sleep. Therefore the solution to sleep problems, I feel, is to identify the causes (there's usually more than one!) and then try to put them right. There's no 'one size fits all' solution. Every one of us is different and we each need to find out what works for us as an individual. Hence I've included a wide variety of tips and techniques in the hope that every reader will find something that helps them to enjoy a better quality of sleep.

Wendy Green

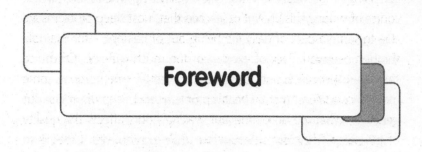

Foreword

by Dr Chris Idzikowski,

Director of the Edinburgh Sleep Centre

The search for a good night's sleep has probably gone on since humanity first appreciated the difference between a good night and a bad night. For many of us that difference hits home after the first child is born. For others, the 'insomniacs', problems with sleep can emerge earlier. The difference between insomniacs and the sleepless is the former often do not know what the cause of their wakefulness is, whereas the latter usually understand the cause. For decades the prescription for both was to apply some potion, tincture, ointment or technique that would bludgeon wakefulness into submission. It's only in the past twenty years or so that we have started to understand the structure of sleep, along with the cycles and rhythms that control it, and how biological treatments fare compared to psychological treatments. We still don't understand how a lot of the alternative and complementary therapies may or may not work – part of the problem being that it is both difficult to fund and do research in this area. Nevertheless, it is helpful to be made aware of the possibilities.

This book is quite the most approachable I have read for a long time. It covers areas that touch on CBT-I (cognitive behavioural therapy for insomnia) without professing to be a book on the subject.

Equally, Wendy Green has provided balance by dealing with areas that are not the subject of 'hard science', for example 'flower power', feng shui, essential oils, etc. (in Chapter 8 – DIY Complementary Therapies). Wendy's coverage of these areas highlights the need for further research on herbal preparations and the effects of nutrition and supplements on sleep.'Notwithstanding, this book helpfully provides a comprehensive rundown of everything that might impact on sleep and help the insomniac.

All in all, it's a fun read in which even the most committed insomniac will find solace on those occasions when they find themselves awake, and out of bed, during the night.

Introduction

Getting an adequate amount of good-quality sleep is vital for your physical, psychological and emotional well-being. According to recent research, 42 per cent of us sleep badly some or most nights, and around a third of people who visit their GP complain about the quality of their sleep. The nation's inability to sleep is estimated to cost the NHS £290 million each year. This book looks beyond short-term fixes such as sleeping pills and offers simple yet effective approaches to dealing with insomnia. But before looking at these, it's important to gain an understanding of sleep and the symptoms of insomnia.

Why is sleep so important?

Research suggests that nearly two thirds of us get less than eight hours sleep and a third sleep for less than six hours. Several long-term studies report that if you sleep less than five hours a night, you're more at risk of developing depression, heart disease, stroke and type 2 diabetes. A recent major study suggested that women who sleep for six hours or less each night were 62 per cent more likely to develop breast cancer than those who sleep seven hours. Lack of sleep has been shown to affect hormones and metabolism, making overeating and weight gain more likely. Some studies suggest that people who don't get enough sleep eat nearly half as much more food as those who do. A hormone called leptin regulates how much we eat, by giving the signal of fullness when we've eaten enough. A hormone called grehlin increases hunger – especially for foods high in carbohydrate. People who sleep poorly have been found to have lower levels of leptin and higher levels of ghrelin, making them more likely to overeat. So ensuring that you get enough sleep can help you to keep your weight in check.

Lack of sleep can lower your immunity, making you more prone to infections. It can also affect your mood, leading to relationship problems. Your co-ordination, reaction times and judgment may be impaired and you're more likely to take risks. All of these factors increase your chances of being involved in road or other accidents – it's estimated that around one in five car accidents are caused by tiredness. Problems sleeping are also linked to unemployment – probably because of poor performance at work and taking time off work through exhaustion; around 15 million of us take days off work because of insufficient sleep. A chronic lack of sleep is also thought to reduce your life expectancy.

Why do we sleep?

Despite the fact that it takes up around one third of our lives, sleep remains a mystery. It's commonly thought that sleep is necessary for the body to rest and recover from the wear and tear of daily life. Yet during sleep the body doesn't actually rest – you're likely to move around between 20 and 40 times each night. And although the body actively restores and repairs tissues during sleep, some studies suggest this can also be carried out whilst relaxing. The brain also remains active during sleep. The main reason that we need to sleep, according to sleep scientists, is because it's necessary for the brain to function efficiently. During sleep the brain processes memories and emotional experiences and the cortex rests and recovers. After just one night without sufficient sleep we are more irritable and less able to deal with pressure. We also find it harder to hold a conversation, work out simple sums and remember things.

Sleep stages

There are two main types of sleep – rapid eye movement (REM) and non-rapid eye movement (NREM). Sleep is also classified in stages. Stages one, two, three and four are NREM sleep and stage five is REM sleep. During sleep you progress through each of these stages, descending from one through to four and then going on into REM sleep. A complete cycle lasts for about 90 minutes. An average adult will have four to six cycles each night.

Each stage lasts for varying periods of time. For example, during the first two cycles, the REM phase is relatively short and sleep stages three and four predominate. Later cycles consist mainly of stage two and REM sleep.

Another factor that affects the length of each stage is age. Around half of a baby's sleep is REM sleep – this will fall gradually until adulthood is reached. An elderly person experiences less stage four sleep.

Stage one – drowsiness

This is the transitional stage between being awake and falling asleep and usually lasts from ten to fifteen minutes. Your brain waves begin to slow down and your muscles start to relax. It's common to experience a falling sensation, followed by a sudden muscle jerk. In a sound sleeper this should only occupy two to five per cent of sleep time.

Stage two – light sleep

At this stage your eye movements stop and your brain waves slow down further, although there are occasional bursts of faster waves, known as sleep spindles. Your heart rate also slows down and your body temperature drops as you sink further into sleep. This stage tends to last around 30 to 40 minutes at a time and takes up around half of the time spent asleep.

Stages three and four – deep sleep

During deep sleep (also known as delta or slow-wave) your brain waves are slow, your blood pressure falls, your breathing slows down and your body temperature falls even lower. Your kidney function is also reduced, so that you produce less urine. In this phase the body releases growth hormone, which has an important role in repairing and maintaining the immune system and body tissues. This is why insufficient deep sleep is commonly thought to have a detrimental effect on the skin, hair and immunity to infections. Some sleep scientists, however, such as Professor Jim Horne, director of Loughborough Sleep Research Centre, argue that the immune system is more likely to be compromised by stress than by lack of sleep and that food and rest are all that's needed for tissue repair.

Slow-wave sleep lasts for up to 40 per cent of total sleep time. It's generally difficult to rouse people from this sleep stage. To be woken by sound, the deeper the sleep, the louder the sound needs to be, or it needs to have some significance for the sleeper. For example, someone whispering the sleeper's name could be enough. If you *are* wakened during this stage, you're likely to feel disorientated and groggy for a while.

Stage five – REM sleep

REM sleep is the period of sleep where the brain is as active as when you are awake and is when you are most likely to dream. It starts after around 60 to 90 minutes of sleep and is characterised by the eyes making quick, darting movements.Your breathing speeds up and your heart rate and blood pressure increase, yet your major voluntary muscles are temporarily paralysed – this may be to prevent you from acting out your dreams and possibly hurting yourself. (People who sleepwalk do so mainly during deep sleep, when those parts of the brain controlling physical actions are still functioning.) REM sleep recurs throughout the night, with the first phase lasting about ten minutes and the last one lasting up to an hour. The total amount of REM sleep per night can be up to two hours – nearly a quarter of the total time asleep.

It's thought that during this phase the brain processes and stores the information gathered during the day, so that it can be retrieved when needed. Dreams are believed to be part of this process, which would explain why insufficient sleep can affect your memory and why you tend to dream about things you experienced or considered that day. This is also when your brain deals with stress and emotions. Though you dream during this stage, it's a lighter type of sleep and not as refreshing as stage four.

Dream on

You can dream at any stage of sleep, but REM dreams are likely to be the most surreal, whilst NREM dreams are likely to relate to more everyday matters.

You spend at least two hours dreaming every night – if you think you don't, it's probably because you simply can't remember your dreams. You're most likely to recall your dreams in the first few minutes after you wake up in the morning. This is because it's easier to remember dreams from REM sleep and most REM sleep takes place in the early hours. But if you don't make a conscious effort to remember, these memories quickly fade.

Research shows that women are better than men at remembering their dreams – especially just before a period, when a woman's body temperature tends to drop. Dreams at this time are usually more intense and therefore make more of an impression. The content of our dreams is unpredictable but is thought to be influenced by our experiences during the day, and even our sleeping environment. For example, a recent study suggested that sleeping in a room smelling of roses led to the participants having pleasant dreams – though not about roses themselves! In other studies, people exposed to unpleasant smells during sleep reported bad dreams. Recent research revealed that older people who have watched black and white television and films are more likely to dream in black and white. Nightmares are more likely to wake you up and tend to have complicated plots (see Chapter 6 – Sleep Disorders).

The sleep/wake cycle

The sleep/wake cycle is governed by the circadian rhythm and the sleep homeostat. The circadian rhythm is like an internal clock that determines when we feel like sleeping and waking. Meal times, exercise patterns and exposure to natural light and darkness can all influence it. The sleep homeostat is a mechanism controlled by brain chemicals, such as melatonin, that ensure you get enough sleep for your body to function. Melatonin production is triggered by darkness and halted by light. Although indoor lighting is weaker than natural light, it can still slow down melatonin production. A typical cycle for most people involves falling asleep between 11 p.m. and midnight and awakening between 6 a.m. and 8 a.m. But differences in circadian rhythms and melatonin production mean some people have more exaggerated sleeping patterns, where they fall asleep and wake up much earlier or later than this.

Are you a lark or an owl?

Do you find yourself falling asleep well before midnight? Are you happy to get up very early and raring to go first thing? If you answered 'yes' to these questions, you're probably what's refered to as a lark. If you answered 'no', then it's likely you're what's known as an owl. Owls tend to prefer going to bed late and getting up later too. They also tend to take a while to get going first thing in the morning.

The average sleep/wake cycle is 24 hours, but can be up to three hours shorter for larks – hence their need to go to bed early. On the other hand, owls can have a much longer daily cycle – up to 28 hours in extreme cases, which explains why they prefer to go to bed and get up later. Our circadian rhythms also seem to be affected by age, with young people tending to be more owl-like and older people becoming more lark-like.

It's important to recognise which end of the spectrum your body clock is in and work with it as much as possible. For example, if you're an owl, it's probably best not to go to bed too early, as you're likely to find it harder to fall asleep. Though of course, most of us have to organise our sleeping patterns to fit in with our working day or other commitments. Owls can help to reset their body clock by getting out in daylight as early in the day as possible. Larks may find that getting out in the daylight late in the afternoon helps them to stay awake longer.

How much sleep do you need?

Evidence suggests that overall, people who sleep less than five hours a night don't live as long as those who sleep seven to eight hours. Paradoxically, sleeping longer than eight hours may also shorten the lifespan. So how long is enough? Research suggests that the idea that eight hours sleep is the norm for healthy adults is a myth and that the average night's sleep for an adult is probably nearer to between seven/seven and a half hours.

However, it seems that individual sleep requirements can vary quite widely, again probably because of differing circadian rhythms, with some people appearing able to function well on as little as four hours' sleep. Age is another factor – babies need up to 18 hours sleep a day and teenagers around nine. Margaret Thatcher famously claimed that she only needed between four and five hours a night whilst she was prime minister – though she did also enjoy one-hour-long power naps during the day! Such individuals are termed 'short sleepers', whilst people who need more than eight hours' sleep are known as 'long sleepers'.

It seems that sleep experts can't agree on whether as a nation we are sleep-deprived or that most of us get an adequate amount of sleep. Sleep expert Dr Neil Stanley believes that around two thirds of us suffer from an inability to enjoy a good night's sleep, and as a result regularly suffer from tiredness and exhaustion during the day. Professor Jim Horne, director of Loughborough University's Sleep Research Centre, claims that this isn't the case – rather than not getting enough sleep, he believes that many of us sleep for too long.

My interpretation is that the answer can be found by listening to your own body. If you're able to fall asleep fairly quickly at night when tired, enjoy largely unbroken sleep and awaken feeling refreshed, then you're probably getting enough sleep – regardless of how much that is. On the other hand, if you regularly find it hard to fall asleep, suffer from broken sleep and awaken the next day feeling groggy and exhausted, you can assume you're not sleeping enough. Dr Neil Stanley seems to agree. He told me: 'We are all different, what is important is that you get the right amount of sleep for you. Simply, if you feel awake and function at a high level during the day, you are probably getting enough sleep, but if on six hours sleep you feel sleepy the next day, then it's not enough for you.' Even Professor Horne concedes: 'The amount of sleep we require is what we need not to be sleepy in the daytime.'

Quick sleep assessment

1. Do you rely on an alarm clock to wake you up?
2. Do you feel sleepy during the day?
3. Do you doze during the day, whenever you have the opportunity?

If you answered 'yes' to any of these questions, it's likely you're sleep-deprived. To find out why you don't get enough sleep, see '1. Identify the root causes of your sleep problems' later in this chapter.

Epworth Sleepiness Scale

The Epworth Sleepiness Scale, devised by a doctor from Melbourne's Epworth Hospital, is a useful tool to help you evaluate your level of daytime sleepiness and help you to decide whether or not you're getting enough sleep. To complete an online version, go to www.nytol.co.uk.

Caught napping?

Some experts argue against napping during the day, claiming that it makes dropping off at night more difficult for some people. However, in many countries, such as Spain and Greece, taking a siesta is the norm. Recent research points to a 37 per cent lower risk of a heart attack in men and women who nap for 30 minutes at least three times a week. The results revealed even greater benefits for working men, with a 64 per cent reduction in risk. Pro-nappers claim that everyone benefits, but especially those suffering from over-tiredness and fatigue due to insufficient sleep at night. Even a 15–20 minute nap can be beneficial.

If you suffer from insomnia only occasionally, taking a short nap shouldn't be a problem, but if you suffer from chronic insomnia, it's probably best to avoid an afternoon snooze so that you can re-establish a regular sleep pattern (see Chapter 4 – Healthy Sleep Habits).

What is insomnia?

In a nutshell 'insomnia' means being unable to sleep. The London Sleep Centre defines it more fully as 'an experience of inadequate or poor quality sleep' with at least one or more of the following: difficulty falling asleep, difficulty maintaining sleep, waking up too early in the morning, non-refreshing sleep.

Insomnia also has daytime repercussions. According to The London Sleep Centre, these include tiredness, lack of energy, difficulty concentrating and irritability.

The different types of insomnia

Insomnia is classified in terms of *when* in the sleep period it's experienced:

Sleep-onset insomnia – this is where you find it hard to *fall* asleep. The average sleeper takes between one and twenty minutes to fall asleep; insomniacs take half an hour, or much longer.

Sleep-maintenance insomnia – this is where you have problems *staying* asleep, i.e. you constantly wake up during the night. Though it's normal to wake up momentarily several times during sleep without even being aware of it, the insomniac lies awake, unable to get back to sleep for several minutes, or even hours at a time. Being awake during the night for half an hour or more is defined by sleep scientists as sleep-maintenance insomnia.

Insomnia is also defined according to how *often* it's experienced:

Transient insomnia – when you have problems sleeping for a few nights.

Short-term insomnia – when you have sleep problems for up to a month.

Chronic insomnia – when you have sleep problems for longer than a month.

According to Dr Neil Stanley, there's another form of insomnia which he has termed 'semisomnia'. He believes that whilst only a few people suffer from chronic insomnia, around two thirds of us sleep poorly most nights, largely because of the stresses and strains of modern life.

Gender differences

Recent research suggests that twice as many women as men suffer from insomnia and it seems that hormonal changes are at least partly to blame. Insomnia is a frequent symptom of premenstrual tension and also often occurs *during* a period when the body temperature goes up, making it harder to fall asleep. Eating foods rich in calcium has been shown to ease premenstrual tension and encourage sleep (see Chapter 5 – Snooze Foods and Supplements).

During pregnancy women are more likely to suffer from disturbed sleep. Usually, this is mainly due to difficulties getting comfortable in bed, as well as the hormonal and brain changes that help to programme the mother-to-be to wake more easily, in preparation for the baby's arrival. In his book *Can't Sleep, Can't Stay Awake: A Woman's Guide to Sleep Disorders* (see Helpful Books) women's sleep disorders specialist Dr Meir Kryger recommends that pregnant women sleep on their side, as this is likely to be the most comfortable position and will increase the flow of blood to the baby. He suggests placing a pillow between the knees to increase the level of comfort – especially for those who don't normally sleep on their sides.

When women go through the menopause they may find that hot flushes disturb their sleep, because they affect the body's temperature control mechanism. Supplements such as black cohosh or red clover and cotton bedding and nightwear can help. Julie Walters explained recently how she'd just started to sleep better after having acupuncture for her insomnia, when the menopause struck. 'At one stage, I was waking up fifteen times a night with flushes. It was deadly because sleep is vital.'

1. Identify the root causes of your sleep problems

Insomnia can be linked to psychological, sleep environment and lifestyle factors, as well as medical conditions, prescribed and recreational drugs and sleep-related disorders. Check the list below – could any of these be contributing to your sleep problems?

Psychological factors – these include stress, anxiety, depression and overstimulation of the brain. Being unrealistic about sleep, i.e. expecting to sleep for a textbook eight hours each night, and underestimating the amount of time you spend asleep, can cause anxiety about sleep and make the problem worse.

The sleep environment – if your bedroom is too hot or too cold, too light, or too noisy, you may have problems falling asleep.

Lifestyle factors – such as a poor diet, exercising too little or too late in the day, lack of daylight and the overuse of stimulants, including coffee, alcohol and nicotine.

Medical conditions – any health problems that can cause breathing difficulties, pain or bladder problems can disrupt your sleep. For example, arthritis, asthma, diabetes, eczema, heart conditions, Parkinson's disease and prostrate problems.

Mental health problems – depression is often linked to early morning waking. Schizophrenia, bipolar disorder and dementia are also linked to sleep disturbances.

Sleep disorders – sleep-related breathing disorders, sleep-related movement disorders, circadian rhythm disorders, parasomnias and hypersomnia can all disrupt sleep.

Medications – including over-the-counter cough medicines and prescribed drugs such as beta blockers, coricosteroids, diuretics and thyroid hormones. Withdrawal from some medications, including antidepressants and sleeping pills, can also lead to sleep problems.

Recreational drugs – such as amphetamines ('speed'), cocaine and ecstasy.

2. Keep a sleep diary

Keeping a sleep diary can also help you to establish the causes of your sleep problems, and it's useful if you decide to seek medical advice. You'll find a sample sleep diary below – you may want to adapt it to suit your own needs. Try to fill it in each day, whilst the details are still fresh in your memory. Remember, the 'time spent awake in bed' will be approximate, because the last thing you need is to feel that you have to watch the clock each night so that you can complete your sleep diary! The downside of keeping a diary is that focussing on your sleep problem could make you even more anxious about it. Try to keep things in perspective and see it as a useful tool to help you assess both your sleep quality and the factors that might be having an impact on it.

Aim to keep a diary for at least a couple of weeks. Hopefully, you should begin to link certain behaviours with poor sleep. For example, a lie-in on a Saturday and Sunday morning may lead to problems falling asleep on Sunday night. Not allowing yourself to wind down before bed might leave you tense and unable to 'switch off' when it's time to go to sleep.

	Day 1	Day 2	Day 3	Day 4
Coffee/tea/alcohol: Quantity? When?				
Drugs: Type? Quantity? When?				
Emotions: e.g. Tense? Anxious?				
Exercise: What? When? How long?				
Food: What? When?				
Bedtime				
Time awake in bed (approx)				
Final wakening time				
Total hours asleep (approx)				
Daytime: Alert/sleepy?				

For a more detailed, printable sleep diary, visit the Patient UK website (see Directory) and enter 'sleep diary' in the search box.

The London Sleep Centre (see Directory) offers an online sleep assessment to help you discover whether you have a sleep disorder.

On the BBC's Science and Nature Website (see Directory) you can find a Sleep Profiler that offers tailored sleep advice based on the answers you give to a short online questionnaire.

Chapter 1

Stress Management

Stress is the way in which our minds and bodies react to responsibilities or pressures that leave us feeling inadequate or unable to cope. It depends on our perception of a situation and our ability to deal with it: a situation that one person finds stressful, another may not.

The brain responds to stress by preparing our body to either stay and face up to the perceived threat, or to run away (known as the 'fight or flight' response). This involves the release of hormones including adrenaline, noradrenaline and cortisol into the bloodstream. As a result the heart rate and breathing patterns speed up and we may sweat. Glucose and fatty acid levels in the blood increase to give us the energy to deal with the threat. Other signs of stress include anxiety, headaches, nausea, reduced appetite or overeating, infections resulting from lowered immunity, heart palpitations and breathlessness.

If the cause of stress is not removed or controlled, cortisol and adrenaline levels remain high, making it hard to wind down at bedtime. Also, people often deal with stress by adopting unhealthy habits, such as smoking, drinking too much alcohol and overeating – all of which can also have a negative impact on sleep patterns. According to Dr Chris Idzikowski, director of the Edinburgh Sleep Centre, stress is one of the causes of insomnia, so it makes sense to prioritise stress management when trying to improve your sleep patterns. Professor Jim Horne suggests that when we are at ease with our lives, good sleep will follow.

3. Work out what makes you stressed

For a couple of weeks note down the situations, times, places and people that make you feel stressed. Next, rate the level of stress they cause from one to ten, with one being a low level of stress and ten signifying extreme stress. Once you've identified your worst stressors look for ways to avoid or minimise them. For example, if driving in rush hour traffic makes you feel especially tense and anxious, see if you can avoid it by going to work slightly earlier or later.

4. Live in the moment

Living in the moment, or practising mindfulness, has been shown to reduce stress levels. It involves giving all of our attention to the here and now, rather than worrying about the past or future, and has its roots in Buddhism. It's based on the philosophy that we can't alter the past, or foretell the future, but we can influence what's happening in our lives right now. By living fully in the present you can perform to the best of your ability, whereas worrying about the past and future can hamper how you function now, and increase stress levels unnecessarily. Living in this way means your experience of life is richer, because instead of doing things on autopilot, all of your senses will be fully engaged in what you are doing. Imagine going for a walk in the park and being so preoccupied with worries about the future that you don't even notice your surroundings. Then think how much more pleasurable and relaxing the experience would be if you took the time to absorb the sights, sounds and smells.

Mindfulness is also about being happy with your life as it is now, rather than thinking you can only be happy when you've achieved certain things – such as a better job, a bigger house, etc. Adopting this attitude towards life will immediately lower your stress levels. If you find it hard to focus on the present, try keeping a daily diary. This will encourage you to think about what's going on in your life now. The best time to do this is at bedtime, as part of your wind-down.

5. Write down your worries and concerns

If anxiety prevents you from sleeping, try writing a list of the things you need to do, or issues that are worrying you and possible solutions. Do this before bedtime, so that you don't lie awake mulling things over when you should be sleeping.

Writing a to-do list will help you avoid feeling overwhelmed. Always prioritise, so that you do the most important and urgent jobs first. You'll feel more in control and organised and you won't forget to do things or miss deadlines. To-do lists work well both at work and at home, helping you to be more efficient and feel less stressed. You're also less likely to lie awake at night making mental lists of tasks you need to do.

A word of caution though – don't feel that you have to complete everything on your list in order to feel less stressed. Inevitably, as you cross off tasks, new ones will replace them. Richard Carlson, author of *Don't Sweat the Small Stuff*, points out that 'the purpose of life *isn't* to get it all done but to enjoy each step along the way' and cautions: 'Remind yourself that when you die, your "in basket" won't be empty.'

6. Reach out to others

Research shows that people who have a good social network tend to enjoy better mental health than those who don't. This may partly be because being able to open up about your problems to someone you can trust helps you to get things into perspective and perhaps find solutions you hadn't thought of. Some research even suggests that social support during stressful periods lowers the level of the stress hormone cortisol in the body. So make time to meet with your family and friends regularly and try to widen your social circle – perhaps by joining a group or class that interests you.

Have a laugh

It's very hard to remain tense whilst laughing. Laughter helps to relieve stress by reducing levels of cortisol and other stress hormones in the body. A good belly-laugh also relaxes the muscles in the upper body. So spend time with people who make you laugh, dig out your favourite comedy, or buy a good joke book and spread a little laughter! The Laughter Network is run by professionals with 'a common goal to bring more laughter and happiness into people's lives'. It offers laughter sessions, classes and workshops across the UK, as well as a Telephone Laughter Club. The website (see Directory) provides more information about the benefits of laughter.

Take a break

Try to schedule regular 'me-time' breaks into your daily routine. Even two fifteen -minute breaks during your working day, when you can do whatever you want, can help to reduce feelings of stress. Something as simple as having a cup of tea and a chat with colleagues or reading the newspaper can have a positive effect, as it can take your mind off your work situation.

7. Go back to nature

Outdoor activities like going to the seaside, going for a walk in the park, visiting the countryside or even just doing a spot of gardening have been shown to improve mood, slow the heart rate, reduce blood pressure and ease muscle tension, making it easier to enjoy a good night's sleep. Experts believe that the higher levels of negative ions near areas with running water, trees and mountains may be partly responsible. Others claim it's down to 'biophilia' – the idea that we have a natural affinity with nature. Research in the Netherlands and Japan suggests that people living near green areas enjoy a longer lifespan and better health than those who live in cities.

8. Enjoy exercise

Exercise helps to reduce stress by enabling the body to put the stress hormones which are triggered by the 'flight or fight' response to good use. Exercise also encourages the release of 'feel good' brain chemicals called endorphins. You don't need to go to the gym to enjoy the benefits of exercise – walking, gardening and even doing household tasks have been shown to offer stress-relieving benefits.

Taking exercise late in the afternoon or early evening will increase your body temperature and metabolism, both of which will drop after about five hours, making you feel drowsy and ready for sleep. Research shows that people who exercise for at least half an hour four times a week sleep around forty minutes longer than those who don't. Insufficient exercise can cause restlessness and sleep problems. Exercise also helps the body to use up stress hormones, which in turn makes it easier to relax and sleep soundly.

9. Learn to relax

Relaxation is the antidote to stress, helping to slow down the breathing and heart rate and calm the mind, making a good night's sleep easier to achieve.

Switch off!

According to research by Dr Neil Stanley, four out of ten of us skip sleep to gain time to do things that seem more important. Many successful, high-achieving people find it particularly difficult to switch off at bedtime, preferring to work into the early hours rather than wind down and go to sleep. Their brain becomes too active to switch off, a condition known as hyperarousal, so that when they do finally go to bed they can't fall asleep. Sleep and energy coach Dr Nerina Ramlakhan believes that hyperarousal is a learned condition that can be unlearned. She suggests that the most important step is to 'recognise that a good night's sleep is essential to your health', then make sure that you give yourself some time to wind down each evening. Try not to work or check your emails after 8 p.m., and switch off your BlackBerry or mobile phone.

Celebrities who can't switch off

Unsurprisingly, several celebrities blame their sleep problems on their inability to switch off at bedtime:

- Matthew Perry, the former *Friends* actor, recently complained that he suffers from chronic insomnia. He revealed that he'd tried comfortable bedding, candles and relaxing music, but that none of these worked. He added, 'It's hard to turn my head off and when I try to go to sleep something creeps in, a little fear, I think.'

- Pop icon Madonna also seems to have problems switching off. She has confessed to sleeping with her BlackBerry under her pillow, in case she remembers something she needs to write down. This may well be why she has reported that she rarely gets more than four hours' sleep each night.

- BBC presenter Jeremy Paxman told recently of how he had suffered from insomnia for over 25 years. He explained: 'I can go to sleep, then I wake up in the middle of the night tossing and turning.' Perhaps his job contributes to the problem – it must be hard to wind down and sleep soundly after taking part in a heated debate on *Newsnight*!

Tune in

When you're feeling wound up and unable to relax before bedtime, try listening to your favourite tunes. There's evidence that taking time out to listen to music you enjoy reduces anxiety, lowers your blood pressure and may even relieve pain through promoting the release of chemicals called endorphins. It might be a good idea to set your iPod/radio on 'sleep timer' so that it turns off after a set amount of time, avoiding the need for you to reach over to switch it off just as you are drifting off.

10. Meditate

Transcendental Meditation (TM) is a simple technique which involves closing your eyes and repeating the same word (mantra) again and again to yourself. When practised daily, TM has been shown to relieve stress, and is thought to reduce insomnia and improve sleep quality. To learn more go to www.t-m.org.uk.

Breathe deeply

Try deep abdominal breathing to help you relax at bedtime. Aim to inhale slowly through your nostrils to a count of three whilst expanding your stomach. Hold for a count of three and then exhale through your mouth, counting to six whilst flattening your stomach. Repeat five times.

Progressive muscle relaxation

This technique, used by many sleep therapists as part of cognitive behavioural therapy (see Chapter 2 – Sleep Psychology), helps to release tension from the muscles and aids sleep. According to Richard Hilliard, director of Relaxation for Living (see Directory), it's impossible to have an anxious mind when your muscles are relaxed.

You can do this in bed to help you drop off, or to help you to go back to sleep if you wake up during the night.

- Take a deep breath and then create tension in your face by clenching your teeth and screwing up your eyes tightly, then relax and breathe out.

- Take a deep breath, then lift the muscles in your shoulders, tense them for a few seconds and then relax, dropping your shoulders and releasing the tension as you breathe out.

- Take a deep breath, then clench your fists and tense the muscles in your arms, hold for a few seconds then release and breathe out.

- Next, tense the muscles in your buttocks and both of your legs, including the thighs and calves, hold, and then release as you breathe out.

- Finally, clench your toes and tense your feet, hold, and then release and breathe out.

The Sleep Council (see Directory) offers a wind-down relaxation routine online.

Chapter 2

Sleep Psychology

Perhaps the main cause of modern sleep problems is the changes in our lifestyles over the past few decades. We live our lives at a faster pace than ever before. We have 24-hour access to televisions and computers for entertainment, shopping and travel. There's less of a distinction between work and home life, with many of us working from home at least some of the time. Our minds are constantly stimulated and consequently many of us can't 'switch off' and fall asleep.

Cognitive behavioural therapy (CBT) has been shown to be very successful in treating insomnia. It targets both the thought processes and behaviours that can lead to sleep problems. For example, in long-term insomnia the brain can start to link your sleep environment with being unable to fall asleep, making sleep ever more elusive. CBT uses psychological strategies to avoid this and ensure that your brain associates your bedroom with sleep (see Chapter 4 – Healthy Sleep Habits).

Your beliefs about sleep, and the lack of it, can cause anxiety and exacerbate sleep problems, so CBT also aims to give you a more realistic view of how much sleep you need and what the effects of insufficient sleep are. In this chapter you'll find some useful techniques to help you adopt new beliefs and thought patterns that encourage sleep. In Chapter 4 – Healthy Sleep Habits, you'll find ideas to help you develop both a bedtime routine and a sleep schedule that will maximise your chances of falling asleep and sleeping through the night.

11. Consider changing your beliefs about sleep

Holding incorrect beliefs about sleep can actually make your insomnia worse, by creating unrealistic expectations and an inaccurate perception of the amount of time you spend lying awake.

For example, many people believe that they need at least eight hours' sleep in order to function, when in fact this may not be the case – everyone has different sleep needs. Professor Jim Horne, director of the Sleep Research Centre at Loughborough University, believes that we can lose a certain amount of sleep without too many problems. He suggests that we can perform well and without feeling tired after around five and a half to six hours sleep, providing that sleep is uninterrupted. He suggests this is because sleep can be divided into two types – 'core' and 'elastic'.

Core sleep lasts for roughly the first four to five hours of sleep and consists of mainly of stages four and five: deep sleep and REM sleep. Professor Horne believes that deep sleep is the most important, because it allows the brain's cortex to recharge and function efficiently the next day. 'Elastic sleep' is made up mainly of stage two, light sleep, which tends to form the latter part of the sleep period. He believes that most people can adapt to having less sleep, so long as they get enough core sleep. He claims that some research shows that the body can cope with less sleep because it can repair itself during time spent relaxing and not just during sleep.

Professor Horne also points out that insomnia sufferers tend to overestimate the amount of time they take to fall asleep; research suggests that few insomniacs take longer than 20 to 30 minutes to fall asleep. He explains that the more a person worries about being unable to drop off, the slower the time spent tossing and turning appears to pass.

Research suggests that insomniacs tend to underestimate the amount of sleep they've had. In one study, chronic insomniacs wore actigraphs – electronic devices that are used to measure sleep. After learning they slept for longer than they'd thought, they began sleeping better.

Studies on sleep deprivation suggest that when we don't get enough sleep, we only need to catch up on about a third of the amount lost, and that the sleep recovered is mainly core stage four and REM sleep.

Below is a list of some commonly held beliefs about sleep. Try reading them and replacing them in your mind with the more realistic ones that follow. With your new perspective on sleep, you should feel less anxious next time you can't drop off or find yourself awake during the night. And you never know, you might even find yourself sleeping better!

Belief: I need eight hours' sleep each night to be healthy and to function properly.
Reality : I may not need eight hours' sleep and can function OK after a poor night's sleep.

Belief: I take one and a half hours to fall asleep at night.
Reality: I probably take about half an hour or less to fall asleep.

Belief: I haven't slept a wink all night.
Reality: Even though I woke up a few times, I've probably slept for at least six hours.

Belief: I didn't sleep well last night, so I'll have to catch up over the next few nights.
Reality: I didn't sleep well last night, but I can catch up with an extra half hour or so.

12. Affirm and sleep

Affirmations have been shown to be useful aids for changing beliefs and behaviours. They are positive statements you make about and to yourself, to help you achieve your goals. An affirmation needs to be personal, so use the word 'I', and it should be positive, so state what you *want* to achieve rather than what you *don't want*.

It's also more effective if you write it as though it's happening now. This imprints a clear image of the result you want to achieve in your subconscious mind, as though you've already achieved it. An effective sleep affirmation would incorporate all of these points. For example, 'I sleep soundly every night.' Repeat your affirmation again and again in your head during the day and at bedtime. Imagine yourself sleeping soundly and feel the energy you'll have after a good night's sleep. Seeing, feeling and hearing your affirmation is thought to make it even more effective. You can also buy CDs with affirmations especially designed to aid sleep (see Useful Products).

13. Calm your racing mind

There's nothing worse than getting into bed feeling exhausted and looking forward to a good night's sleep, only to find that your mind simply won't switch off. Following a relaxing bedtime routine to help you 'put the day to bed' and writing down any thoughts or worries should help you to avoid this problem, but when this isn't enough, try these techniques.

Professor Colin A. Espie, director of the University of Glasgow Sleep Research Laboratory and author of *Overcoming Insomnia and Sleep Problems*, recommends the word 'the' as an effective thought-blocking tool. He suggests repeating 'the' in your head every two seconds for up to five minutes. He claims that doing this helps you to disconnect from both the outside world and your own thought processes, because on its own 'the' has no meaning and doesn't spark any emotion except, hopefully, boredom!

Sleep expert Dr Neil Stanley recommends listening to soft music, or thinking of a peaceful setting – real or imaginary.

14. Use visualisation to help you sleep

Using visualisation to help empty the mind and induce sleep is nothing new – we've been 'counting sheep' for over a century. The following sleep visualisation is designed to ease you into a more relaxed state, to allow you to drift off to sleep more easily.

Stairway to sleep

1. Imagine standing at the top of a beige-carpeted staircase with ten candle-lit steps.

2. Start walking slowly down the stairs, counting each step, from ten down to zero.

3. Feel each step leading you into deeper and deeper levels of relaxation.

4. By the time you reach the bottom step you are ready to drift off to sleep...

15. Cast aside your worries

Problems that seem insignificant during the day can seem insurmountable in the middle of the night. You might have been asleep, but suddenly you find yourself wide awake, mulling over something that's going on in your life. Your mind goes into overdrive, trying to think of a solution, but there just doesn't seem to be one. When this happens, I've found that what works for me is to tell myself firmly, 'You can't do anything about this now, so go to sleep and worry about it tomorrow.' It might help if you imagine your worries are inside a helium balloon, then visualise letting go of the balloon and watching it, and your worries, float away.

16. Stop trying to sleep

So you've been trying to fall asleep for what seems like ages: you've tried muscle relaxation, affirmations and visualisations, but you just can't seem to drift off. What can you do? You could try getting out of bed and only returning when you feel sleepy (see Chapter 4 – Healthy Sleep Habits). But if you find this unappealing, or you've tried doing this without success, there's another ploy you can try. According to Dr Chris Idzikowski, director of the Edinburgh Sleep Centre, for the insomniac *trying* to sleep is counterproductive. So perhaps the simplest solution, when all else has failed, is to remind yourself that the world won't end if you don't sleep for seven or eight hours tonight and then... *stop trying to sleep*!

Chapter 3

Sleep Sanctuary

To promote healthy sleep, your bedroom needs to be a space that you associate with rest and sleeping. This chapter gives tips on ways you can make your bedroom comfortable and inviting – somewhere you can relax and enjoy falling asleep and waking up.

17. Make your bedroom a peaceful haven

The sound of silence

Noise can disturb sleep, especially REM sleep, and most people sleep more soundly and find it easier to drop off in a quiet environment. In studies, traffic noise has been shown to increase the time it takes to fall asleep. Double glazing can go a long way towards blocking out traffic and other outside noises. Earplugs can also help – especially if your partner or a family member snores – and are widely available in pharmacies. For more information on snoring and how you and your partner/family member can deal with it see Chapter 6 – Sleep Disorders.

'White noise', such as the sound of the ocean, can be used to filter out background noise and encourage slower brain waves, thus improving sleep quality. Studies have suggested that white noise can help babies aged one week to two years to fall asleep more quickly. Another study that involved playing ocean sounds to patients recovering from heart bypasses, following their transfer from intensive care, suggested that they slept more soundly than patients who weren't exposed to white noise. Various white noise products are available (see Useful Products). However, these won't help everyone – some people (myself included) find that *any* noise disrupts their sleep.

Avoid sleep stealers

It's best not to keep a television in the bedroom – watching TV last thing at night can overstimulate the brain, making it difficult to switch off. Likewise, it's best not to use a computer late at night, as it can have a similar effect. The bright lights from TV and computer screens can also interfere with the production of the hormones that regulate the sleep/wake cycle.

Blackout

Choose heavy, dark-coloured curtains to ensure your bedroom is as dark as possible. Line your curtains with blackout cloth, or invest in some blackout blinds. Darkness stimulates your brain to produce the sleep hormone melatonin; light can disrupt this process. As you wind down before bedtime it might help if you dim the lights.

18. Keep your cool

Your brain tries to reduce your body temperature at night to slow down your metabolism and conserve energy. So to encourage sleep, keep your room fairly cool (around 16 °C) and airy – most people keep their bedroom too warm. Cotton nightwear and bedding are best for helping you to maintain a steady temperature, because cotton absorbs sweat.

If hot flushes wake you at night, sleep with a cotton sheet under the duvet. When a flush strikes, you can throw the duvet off and still have a light cover over you. If you suffer from cold feet in bed, wearing socks might help to improve your sleep. Just before you fall asleep your body tends to redistribute heat from your core to your extremities, so keeping your feet warm could induce sleep. Professor Jim Horne advises keeping the feet warm and the face cool – a practice he says many people find helps them to fall asleep.

19. Choose a suitable bed and bedding

We spend around a third of our lives in our beds, yet most of us pay little attention to whether or not they're supportive, comfortable and sleep-enhancing. The Sleep Council suggests that if you wake up with aches and pains which disappear during the day, you are not sleeping as well as you did previously, and/or if your mattress shows signs of wear, it's probably time to change your bed. Generally, you should replace your bed at least every eight years.

Choosing a bed

The two main types of bed base are bedsteads and divans. Divans are the most popular option, but bedsteads have enjoyed a revival recently.

Divans are available in four main types:

Sprung-edge divans – these have an open coil or pocket spring base on a frame. They provide even support and shock absorption, increasing the life of the mattress, and are the most luxurious option.

Solid or platform top divans – these have a non-sprung top panel, usually made from hardboard, and are firmer and cheaper than sprung bases.

Firm-edge divans – these have fewer, bigger, heavy-duty springs, with a solid wooden-sided frame.

Flexible-slatted divans – these have flexible soft wood slats that make them slightly springy.

Bedsteads can have either flexible/rigid wooden slats or flexible/rigid wire mesh to support the mattress.

It's thought we lose around half a pint of moisture each night through perspiration, and the resulting change in temperature and thirst can increase waking during the night. Some experts recommend wooden-slatted bedsteads for uninterrupted sleep, because they allow air to circulate beneath the mattress, helping to disperse body heat and reduce sweating. Bedsteads tend to be more hardwearing than divan bases, so you may be able to just replace the mattress after eight years, rather than the entire bed.

You can also buy adjustable bases that allow the user to raise the head or foot of the bed, which can be helpful for various complaints. For example, sleeping with your head raised can reduce snoring, whilst sleeping with the feet raised can alleviate back pain and improve circulation. Raising the head of the bed can also make getting in and out of it easier.

Always buy the biggest bed you can afford. If you share a bed with a partner, you need to make sure there's enough space so that the other person can sleep soundly when one of you has a restless night.

The Sleep Council (see Directory) is sponsored by bed manufacturers, but nevertheless offers lots of useful advice on buying a bed. To prevent back pain, they recommend that you choose a supportive, rather than a hard bed, cautioning that an orthopaedic or firmer bed is not always the best option and that often a medium firm bed with proper cushioning is better. The website offers an online Bed MOT to help you to decide whether or not you need to change your bed, as well as a Bed Profile Questionnaire and Bed Buyers Guide to help you work out what type of bed would best suit your needs and circumstances.

Choosing a mattress

As a rule of thumb, mattresses should be changed as soon as they start to sag, or become uncomfortable and lumpy, or when they're eight years old. If your bed base is still in good condition, you could opt to just replace the mattress. Research by Dr Chris Idzikowski, director of the Edinburgh Sleep Centre, indicated that a new mattress could, on average, extend sleep by 42 minutes.

A common question is whether a hard or a soft mattress is best for your back. Dr Chris Idzikowski warns that a hard mattress may offer support, but it can be uncomfortable, as contact with the body is limited – leading to undue pressure and pain in those areas. On the other hand, a soft mattress offers more body contact, but it may sag and offer inadequate support.

Physiotherapist Sammy Margo, author of *The Good Sleep Guide*, agrees. She advises that super-firm mattresses aren't necessarily a good thing and suggests that you should choose a mattress that moulds to your body and supports you, so there's no undue pressure anywhere. The one that suits you is dependent on things like your weight – the heavier you are the firmer your mattress needs to be – and your body shape; women have more body contours and are more comfortable on a softer mattress, whereas men tend to prefer a firmer mattress. However, when you're buying a mattress for yourself and a partner you'll probably need to find one that suits you both – or consider two single mattresses on a super king-size base.

Too hard or too soft?

An easy way to check whether a mattress gives you the right support is to lie on your back and slip a hand under your lower back. There should be just enough space for your hand to fit in the gap between your back and the mattress. If there's no space, the mattress is probably too soft. If there's a lot of space, it's likely that it is too hard for you.

Which mattress?

The two main types of mattress are sprung and non-sprung. Sprung mattresses are built around coils or springs. The more springs in the mattress, the more support it will give.

Non-sprung mattresses can be constructed from a variety of fillings including latex, cotton, coir, wool or foam. Memory foam is a fairly recent innovation that's claimed to mould to your shape and provide superior comfort and support.

If a new bed or mattress is out of the question, you can try adapting your current mattress. If your mattress is sagging or too soft, try placing a board in between it and the base of the bed. If your mattress is too firm, or just worn, try covering it with a mattress topper – you can buy them made from memory foam, polyester, duck down or feathers.

Picking a pillow

Choosing the right pillow can make a huge difference to the quality of your sleep. The right pillow will provide support for the neck and head and keep your spine in line with your neck.

You should consider your favoured sleeping position when choosing a pillow. If you like to sleep on your stomach, The Sleep Council advises using a soft pillow, and Sammy Margo suggests it should be fairly flat, to keep the spine and neck aligned. If you prefer lying on your side, choose a medium-soft one. If you tend to sleep on your back, you need a firm pillow. The best pillow height for you also depends on the width of your shoulders – for narrow shoulders choose a flatter pillow; if you have broad shoulders, you may need two pillows. If you have neck or back problems, it may be best to talk to a physiotherapist, who should be able to recommend a pillow that best suits your needs.

There are numerous types of pillow fillings. Down and feather are comfortable and luxurious, but may not be suitable if you suffer from asthma or allergies. Cotton fillings are available in various thicknesses and are ideal for those with allergies. Foam-filled pillows tend to be cheaper, but may not offer as much comfort.

According to Sammy Margo, if your pillow is six months old or more it could need replacing. With normal wear and tear you can expect a polyester pillow to last for six months to two years; a down pillow should last around five years and a feather pillow about eight years. If at any time your pillow shows signs of losing its shape, it's probably time to buy a new one.

Sammy suggests testing the support of down and feather pillows by laying the fluffed up pillow on a hard surface. Next, fold it in half, squeezing out the air. Then release the pillow – if it returns to its original position it's still supportive, but if it remains folded, it's time to replace it. To check the support of a polyester pillow do the same – but this time place an object weighing about 300 g (for example, a trainer) on top. A pillow that's still supportive will unfold itself and throw off the object – one that stays folded needs replacing.

Buying bedding

Your choice of bedding will largely depend on your budget and what you find the most comfortable. Cotton sheets and pillowcases are popular because cotton feels cool and fresh and absorbs sweat. Brushed cotton (flannelette) feels warmer, making it more comfortable in the winter. Polyester bedding is usually the cheapest, but is less breathable and absorbent. Linen bedding feels especially light, cool and comfortable, but it's expensive. Silk sheets and pillow cases, though expensive, are extremely soft and luxurious and are claimed to stop your skin from creasing and drying out during the night.

Duvets can be filled with synthetic materials such as polyester or natural materials such as feather and/or down. Natural fillings hold warmth better and allow your skin to breathe during sleep, but again, may not be suitable if you suffer from asthma or allergies. They also need to be professionally cleaned. Synthetic duvets are usually much cheaper than natural ones and can often be washed in a domestic washing machine, making them easier to care for. Polyester microfibre is made to feel more like natural fillings and, though more expensive, duvets filled with it are bulkier and more cosy.

You could opt for a lightweight summer (3–4.5 tog), a spring/ autumn weight (7.0–10.5 tog) and a winter weight (12.0–3.5 tog) duvet, that you can swap around according to the seasons. It's often cheaper and easier to buy a duvet set that contains both a summer and spring/autumn weight duvet that can be used individually or buttoned together to make a winter weight duvet.

For more tips on making your bedroom conducive to sleep, see '45. Feng shui your bedroom' in Chapter 8 – DIY Complementary Therapies.

Chapter 4
Healthy Sleep Habits

There's a lot of evidence that we can improve our sleep patterns by adopting certain habits and routines during our waking hours. This chapter looks at how getting outdoors, being active and following a bedtime routine can all help to improve sleep. It also examines how scheduling your sleep can help to regulate your body clock and encourage your brain to associate your bed with sleep. Travelling abroad by plane and working shifts can disrupt sleep patterns: I've included practical tips that can help to restore sleep in those situations.

20. Get out more

Spending time outdoors during the day can help you sleep better at night. Exposure to sunlight stops your brain producing the sleep hormone melatonin, making it easier for your body to produce the hormone at night, which helps you to fall asleep more easily and sleep more soundly. Being in natural sunlight also raises the levels of serotonin (the hormone your body converts into melatonin) which boosts both mood and the ability to deal with stress. Remember, when spending time in the sun, that you should stay in the shade from 11 a.m. to 3 p.m. and use factor 30+ sunscreen to prevent your skin from burning.

21. Follow a bedtime routine

In his report, 'Making time For Sleep', Dr Neil Stanley recommends that we spend time preparing for sleep, both physically and mentally, before bedtime and view sleep as a pleasurable activity. He claims that six out of ten adults don't regularly wind down before bedtime.

Try to establish a bedtime routine that suits you and helps you to unwind. It could include having a warm bath, dimming the lights, sipping a warm, milky drink and perhaps spending a few minutes reading a good book, or listening to relaxing music, before taking to your bed. Watching TV is OK, so long as it helps you to let go of the stresses and strains of your day. (Although most experts advise against having a TV in the bedroom as it detracts from the brain learning to associate the bedroom with sleep.) Reducing the level of light you're exposed to in the evening helps to ease your body into sleep mode by encouraging the production of the sleep hormone melatonin. A dimmer switch is ideal for this, or try winding down by lamp, or candlelight.

Taking a warm, but not hot, bath before bed can also aid sleep. The warmth relaxes the muscles and mind and raises your temperature slightly. The subsequent drop in temperature when you get out of the bath gives your body the 'message' that it's time for sleep.

Your brain will eventually become programmed to associate these events with sleep, making it easier for you to drop off. Sticking to a regular bedtime also helps to train your brain to expect sleep at that time.

Bedtime story

Many people find that reading in bed helps them to drop off to sleep. Sleep experts are divided on whether reading in bed is a good idea. Some, such as Professor Colin A. Espie, argue that it may interfere with your brain associating your bed with sleep. Dr Neil Stanley suggests that everyone is different and that if you find reading in bed helps you to drop off, then you should do it. However, it's probably best to avoid thrillers or horror stories, as these may overstimulate the brain, making it harder to fall asleep!

22. Stick to a sleep schedule

Sticking to a regular sleep schedule has been found to be a successful strategy to help treat insomnia. Drastically changing your sleep patterns confuses the body clock and affects the quality of your sleep, whereas going to bed and getting up at roughly the same time each day helps your body clock to function properly, making it easier to fall asleep. You can however experiment with the number of hours you spend in bed to determine the length of time that leads to the best sleep quality.

23. Restrict your time in bed

If you spend a lot of your time in bed awake and unable to sleep, try cutting the number of hours you spend there, until you begin to sleep for a higher proportion of your time in bed. This helps your brain to associate your bed with sleep, rather than with being awake. First, you need to work out roughly how many hours you sleep each night, on average – consult your sleep diary if you keep one. Next, you need to decide what time you want to get up – this obviously needs to fit in with your work, or other commitments. So, for example, if you find that you tend to sleep only about six hours out of the eight you spend in bed and need to get up at 7 a.m. each morning, you should go to bed at 1 a.m. If you sleep less than five hours, you should aim to spend five hours in bed each night. You must then follow this schedule every night – even at weekends. The aim is for you to establish a regular sleep pattern.

Try to follow your natural sleep patterns – if you're a lark set your bedtime fairly early, with an early rising time; if you're an owl, it will probably work better if you go to bed and get up later.

Gradually increase your time in bed

Once you've slept for about 90 per cent of the time you spend in bed for a full week (for example, if you spend six hours in bed and are sleeping for about five and a half hours), you can start to gradually increase the amount of time you spend in bed. Professor Colin A. Espie recommends either going to bed 15 minutes earlier or getting up 15 minutes later. Again, once you find yourself sleeping for about 90 per cent of your time in bed for a week you can increase it by another 15 minutes, until eventually you reach the point where you're sleeping for as long as you need. This process might sound laborious, but research suggests that it is effective in the long term.

Sleep restriction: case studies

Freelance writer and editor Joy Persaud recently revealed how sleep restriction helped her to overcome her five-year struggle with insomnia. She described how she hadn't enjoyed a full night's sleep for years and spent her nights feeling increasingly distressed about her wakefulness and her days feeling permanently exhausted. Sometimes she managed to get four hours' sleep spread across the night and other times she'd only drop off half an hour before her alarm clock went off.

After she nearly crashed her car twice in one day, Joy's partner booked her an appointment at the London Sleep Centre. Following an initial consultation and a monitored sleep at the centre, she was diagnosed with bruxism (teeth grinding) and periodic limb movement (involuntary limb movements) which were making it difficult for her to achieve deep sleep. Her treatment included a strict sleep regimen that involved going to bed and getting up at the same time each day. Her waking time was determined by the earliest time she needed to get up – which was 6.45 a.m. – and her bedtime was set at any time after midnight. Early nights, naps and lie-ins weren't allowed. She was also advised to avoid chocolate, alcohol and caffeine and was prescribed a muscle relaxant for a year, to deal with the teeth grinding and involuntary limb movements, as well as melatonin to help regulate her sleep cycle. Exercise was encouraged, to use up adrenaline released through stress and release endorphins – 'feel good' chemicals that help to improve sleep quality.

At first she reported feeling 'like a zombie' and wanting to go to bed before midnight, but nine months after her diagnosis she noted that she was sleeping for between six and seven hours a night. Four months later she was still averaging six to seven hours sleep a night and still trying to go to bed and wake up at 'roughly the same time every day'. If she did wake up, she was able to fall asleep again within a few minutes. She had found the regime 'shockingly difficult' but, thanks to the support of her loved ones, it had worked. She concluded: 'Now when someone says "sleep well", I think to myself: I will.'

Lynda Brown, author of *The Insomniac's Best Friend: How to Get a Better Night's Sleep*, tried sleep restriction and found that it worked really well for her, gradually enabling her to fall asleep without difficulty most nights and to get a 'good chunk of sleep'. She warns that it's common to feel drowsy at first and that it takes two to four weeks to feel an improvement. Initially you may be getting, or feel as though you're getting, less sleep, but eventually you will begin to sleep more deeply and awaken feeling more refreshed.

John Wiedman, author of *Desperately Seeking Snoozin': The Insomnia Cure From Awake to Zzzz*, also found that sleep restriction, along with a pre-sleep routine and relaxation techniques, helped him to beat his chronic insomnia. After a decade of often managing only a couple of hours of poor-quality sleep he found that, after spending ten weeks following his new regime, he was able to sleep for seven and a half hours most nights.

24. Only go to bed when you're sleepy

Although you've identified your ideal bedtime, it's important that you only go to bed when you feel sleepy-tired. If you go to bed feeling wide-awake, you're unlikely to fall asleep for a while, or you may wake up early. In his book, *Overcoming Insomnia and Sleep Problems*, Professor Colin A. Espie cautions that you need to be aware of the difference between feeling tired and feeling sleepy-tired. He explains that feeling tired doesn't necessarily mean that you will be able to fall asleep, whereas feeling sleepy is your body's signal that you're ready for sleep. Signs of sleepiness usually include watery or itchy eyes, yawning, feeling drained, achy muscles and having problems keeping your eyes open. Following a bedtime routine that helps you to wind down should help you to feel sleepy. If you don't feel sleepy enough when it's your bedtime, find something relaxing to do, and preferably avoid bright lighting.

Don't clockwatch

If you wake during the night, avoid looking at the clock, as you may start worrying about how long you have left to sleep and this might hinder you from dropping off again. Instead, keep your eyes shut and try deep breathing to ease yourself back to sleep.

25. Get up if you can't sleep

If you can't fall asleep within what you feel is about 20 minutes of going to bed or waking up during the night, most sleep experts advise that you should get up and go into another room. I personally find this hard, but sometimes it is better than tossing and turning and worrying about your lack of sleep.

Try drinking a glass of milk and doing something that relaxes you – such as reading a book or listening to soft music, but avoid watching TV or using the computer or anything that might overstimulate you brain. Popular British cook Nigella Lawson has said that she often sits up copying out recipes when she can't sleep – little wonder that she describes herself as a 'long-time insomniac'.

Only return to your bed when you feel sleepy again – this will help to strengthen your brain's connection between your bed and sleep.

26. Sleep better when working shifts

Those who work during the night often find they have problems sleeping during the day; daytime noises, daylight and the body's own circadian rhythms all contribute to the difficulties. These tips may help.

- Try to have just one block of sleep.
- Use black-out curtains or blinds, or an eye mask, to encourage production of the sleep hormone melatonin.
- Wear earplugs to block out daytime noises.
- Unplug your landline telephone and switch off your mobile, or turn it on to silent mode.
- A US company called Circadian offers specialist advice for shift workers – see the Directory for more details.

27. Prevent jet lag

One of the downsides of long-distance journeys is that high-speed travel to a different time zone confuses your body clock and can adversely affect your sleep patterns – a condition known as jet lag. Other symptoms include fatigue and disorientation. These steps have been shown to help minimise the effects of jet lag.

- Change your watch to your destination time as soon as you board the plane, to help you mentally adjust.
- Eat after you land, rather than on the plane, to help your body clock adjust.
- When you arrive at your destination, try not to sleep until it is bedtime in that time zone.
- If it's bedtime when you arrive, follow your usual bedtime routine to encourage sleep.
- Dehydration is thought to make jet lag worse, so drink plenty of water and avoid alcohol during your flight.
- Get out in the daylight as much as possible.
- Be as active as you can during the day.

Dr Chris Idzikowski has developed a jet lag calculator that offers tailored advice to help you minimise jet lag – go to www.britishairways.com/travel/drsleep/public/en_gb.

Chapter 5

Snooze Foods and Supplements

What you eat and drink can have a direct effect both on how quickly you drop off and how soundly you sleep. Substances found in foods can promote or prevent sleep and a lack of certain nutrients can contribute to insomnia. Eating a balanced diet will help to promote well-being and sound sleep: in this chapter I've given guidelines on how to achieve this and have also included information about supplements that may aid sleep.

Vitamin and mineral supplementation is controversial; some experts argue that we should obtain essential nutrients in their natural form and that vitamin supplementation can be dangerous, whereas nutritional therapists like Patrick Holford, founder of the Institute of Optimum Nutrition, claim that supplementation can add years to people's lives. Some argue that many people don't eat sufficient fresh food and that even when they do, these foods may be low in nutrients due to the poor quality of the soil they were grown in and the length of time spent in storage and transportation. My feelings are that we should all aim to eat a healthy balanced diet, but when a busy lifestyle or illness means this isn't possible, vitamin and mineral supplementation can help to prevent deficiencies.

Note:

Care needs to be taken with the fat soluble vitamins A, D and K, as any excess amounts are stored in the liver and can be harmful.

28. Balance your blood sugar

Eating in a way that helps to keep your blood sugar steady during the daytime will help to ensure that your sleep isn't disrupted by hunger.

Don't stuff or starve

Try not to overeat near bedtime, as it may cause you discomfort and prevent you from sleeping soundly. It's also likely to cause a surge in body temperature, making it hard to fall asleep. Likewise, don't eat too little – your body needs nutrients to repair itself and hunger pangs may keep you awake, or wake you during the night.

Eat low GI foods

The glycaemic index (GI) indicates the rate by which a food raises the level of sugar in the blood. Carbohydrates with a high GI include refined foods such as white bread, pastries, biscuits, cakes, sweets and fizzy drinks, which are easily converted into glucose and cause your blood sugar to rise rapidly. Carbohydrates with a low GI, such as multigrain bread, porridge, sweet potatoes, wholewheat pasta and brown rice, contain fibre, so they take longer to digest. This means the glucose is released more slowly, keeping your blood sugar steady, which makes you feel full for longer and less likely to be woken by a rumbling tummy during the night.

For a low GI diet, as well as eating these slow-release carbohydrates, you need to include lots of fruits, vegetables, beans and low-fat dairy products such as yogurt, skimmed/semi-skimmed milk and cheese. You should also eat small amounts of nuts, fish and lean meat. Leave the skins on potatoes to keep their GI low – eating potatoes without the skin enables the glucose to be digested more quickly. New potatoes boiled in their skins have the lowest GI.

29. Be a tryptophan fan

Bananas are suitable for bedtime snacking because they are rich in tryptophan, an amino acid that the body uses to make serotonin. Interestingly, low levels of serotonin are linked to depression, of which insomnia can be a symptom. Not only is serotonin calming – the body also uses it to make the sleep-inducing hormone melatonin. Other foods rich in tryptophan include chicken, turkey, dairy foods, eggs, beans, rice, oats, nuts, seeds, dates, hummus and wholegrains.

Sleepy suppers

A carbohydrate-rich meal increases the brain's uptake of tryptophan. So an evening meal containing brown rice or pasta with chicken or turkey and a green vegetable would help ensure a good night's sleep. If you are hungry just before bedtime, a light snack, such as a handful of nuts or seeds, wholemeal pitta bread with hummus, wholegrain cereal with skimmed milk or wholegrain crisp breads with a little peanut butter could promote sound sleep.

Both the Egyptians and the Romans recognised that lettuce helped to induce sleep. It has a sedative effect, because it contains a substance called lactucarium, which has a similar effect to opium. Try adding it to a chicken or turkey sandwich. The Sleep Council recommends a 'sleep sandwich' of bananas, marmite and lettuce, to promote sound sleep. This combination would also be rich in tryptophan and B vitamins, but having never tried it I can't vouch for the taste!

The Egyptians ate onions to aid relaxation and sleep. They contain quercetin, a plant pigment with mild sedative properties. Red and yellow varieties of onions contain the most quercetin. Try adding them to evening meals like stir-fries, curries, casseroles and broths.

Include chilli in your evening meal. According to a study published in *The New Scientist*, the capsaicin they contain helps to regulate your sleep cycle, allowing you to fall asleep more easily and wake up feeling more refreshed. However, don't overdo it – some people find that eating too much chilli can lead to stomach upsets.

30. Eat magnesium-rich foods

Magnesium is often known as 'nature's tranquiliser'. Lack of magnesium has been linked to early morning waking. In her book *Let's Eat Right to Keep Fit*, the late renowned American nutritonist Adelle Davis linked insufficient magnesium to insomnia. The well-known nutritional therapists Patrick Holford and Ian Marber also advocate a magnesium-rich diet for sound sleep. Marber describes magnesium as a 'fantastic relaxant' that 'enables the body to deal more effectively with stress', adding, 'so if your mind is working overtime then this is the mineral for you'. Holford warns that your magnesium levels are likely to be low if you eat a lot of sugary foods, or are particularly stressed. As well as calming the mind, magnesium helps to relax the muscles and prevent night cramps.

The recommended daily intake is 270 mg for men and 300 mg for women. To ensure an adequate intake of magnesium in your diet eat plenty of dark green leafy vegetables (such as spinach, broccoli and kale) seafoods, tomato puree, nuts, seeds, wholegrains, beans (including baked beans), peas, potatoes, oats and yeast extract. Avoid drinking too much alcohol – drinking more than the recommended 14 units a week for women and 21 units for men can affect magnesium absorption. Fizzy drinks are also best avoided, because the phosphates they contain interfere with magnesium absorption.

31. Get your calcium quota

Calcium has also been linked to improved sleep. Adelle Davis warned that 'calcium deficiency often shows itself as insomnia, another form of an inability to relax'. The richest sources of calcium are dairy foods – especially low-fat milk, hard cheese, edam and yogurt. Tinned sardines are also a good source – if you eat the bones. Good non-animal calcium providers include green leafy vegetables such as kale and purple broccoli, watercress, leeks, parsnips, figs, dates, dried apricots, oats, lentils, beans, Brazil nuts, almonds, seeds, tofu and soya.

To increase your absorption of the calcium they contain, sprinkle leafy green vegetables with a little ordinary vinegar. Drinking a tablespoon of cider vinegar and honey in warm water once or twice a day is also recommended for promoting calcium absorption.

'Good' bacteria – probiotics such as *Lactobacillus* – seem to improve calcium absorption. There are various probiotic foods and drinks available, but they can be expensive – natural live bio-yogurt is a good, relatively cheap source.

Eating prebiotic foods such as onions, tomatoes, leeks, garlic, cucumber, celery and bananas, which feed and encourage the growth of probiotics in the gut, could also help. Don't forget, calcium is found in water – especially in hard water areas and some bottled waters.

Note:

It's recommended that your daily calcium intake doesn't exceed more than 2,000–2,500 mg. A higher intake may interfere with the absorption of other minerals, such as iron, and could lead to other problems.

Interestingly, women are more likely to suffer from insomnia just before a period and eating a calcium-rich diet seems to help PMT symptoms.

32. Eat foods containing B vitamins

An adequate intake of the B vitamins is essential for a healthy nervous system – and sound sleep. All B vitamins are involved in the control of tryptophan, whilst B6 promotes the production of calming serotonin and B12 boosts the effects of sleep-inducing melatonin. A balanced diet containing animal proteins (e.g. meat, milk, eggs and cheese), wholegrains, yeast extract, green vegetables and nuts should supply enough B vitamins for most people's needs. If you're a vegan, or you eat a lot of processed foods, you may be lacking in these B vitamins. Also, if you're under stress, your body's requirements for these nutrients shoot up. If you suffer from long-term insomnia and feel you might not be getting enough of these vitamins, it may be worth trying a vitamin B-complex supplement.

33. Boost your iron intake

Iron deficiency is often linked to restless leg syndrome, which is a fairly common sleep disruptor. Good sources of iron include salmon, sardines, tuna, eggs, liver, meat, poultry, dark green leafy vegetables, fortified breakfast cereals, wholemeal bread, nuts and dried fruits, such as prunes and apricots. Iron absorption is improved by vitamin C, so try to have vegetables, fruit or fruit juice with your meals.

34. Sip and sleep

It's best not to drink large quantities of any liquid near bedtime, to avoid waking to make trips to the bathroom.

Having said that, a warm milky drink makes a great nightcap. Not only does milk contain tryptophan, it also contains calcium, to soothe and relax. Semi-skimmed or skimmed milk are best because they contain less fat, which means they place less of a burden on the digestive system during sleep. Add a vanilla pod and a little honey for a delicious, relaxing bedtime drink.

Nightcap

Alcohol is normally not recommended at bedtime if you have problems sleeping. Although it has a relaxing effect, helping you to fall asleep, it's also a stimulant, so you're more likely to wake up during the night and less likely to enter the deeper stages of sleep – especially if you drink more than the recommended daily limit of two to three units for women and three to four units for men. It also has diuretic (urination increasing) properties, so you could wake up to make trips to the toilet. But it's thought that just one glass of Cabernet Sauvignon, Merlot or Chianti at bedtime can help you sleep more soundly, because these wines contain grape skins that are rich in the sleep hormone melatonin.

Soothing chamomile

Drinking chamomile tea is a well-known antidote to insomnia. Chamomile flowers contain the amino acid glycine, which is a muscular and nerve relaxant, and there is some scientific evidence that they may help to induce sleep. Chamomile tea bags are widely available, or you can make your own tea. Chamomile can be grown in a sunny spot, in pots or in the garden. Pick the flowers whilst in full bloom and hang them upside down in small bunches in a well-ventilated warm room until they are crisp and completely dry. Store the dried flowers in an airtight jar. To make up a cup of tea, pour boiling water over one tablespoon of the dried flowers, cover and leave to stand for five to ten minutes. Strain, add honey to taste and drink whilst hot. Chamomile tea has a distinctive, apple-like flavour.

If you dislike the taste, try adding two or three bags to a hot bath to enjoy the benefits without having to drink the tea.

Lemon balm calm

Lemon balm (*Melissa officinalis*), so called because of its lemon-scented leaves, has soothing and calming properties, making it an ideal bedtime supplement – either as a tea, or in a proprietary sleep preparation (see below). The herb is approved for 'nervous sleeping disorders' by Commission E of the German Federal Institute for Drugs and Medical Devices. Commission E is the German governmental agency that assesses the safety and effectiveness of herbal products.

Lemon balm can be grown in a sunny or part-shaded spot in a large pot or in the garden and needs well-drained soil. Pour boiling water over one tablespoon of fresh (or one teaspoon of dried) herb, leave to brew for five to ten minutes, then strain, sweeten to taste with honey and drink whilst hot. If you don't like herbal teas, try adding finely chopped leaves to fish or meat dishes. They also taste great blended into a melon or pear smoothie.

35. Avoid foods containing tyramine

Tyramine is an amino acid that encourages the release of norepinephrine, a brain chemical that has a stimulant effect on the body and may interfere with sleep in some individuals. If you think you might be affected, try to avoid eating foods containing tyramine in the evening. These include the nightshade family of vegetables, i.e. potatoes, tomatoes, courgettes, aubergines and spinach. Tyramine is also found in aged or fermented foods such as beers, tinned meats, mature cheeses, salami, pepperoni and yeast extract.

36. Curb your coffee drinking

The BBC sport presenter, Gaby Roslin, recently commented that sleep was the best 'beauty fix', adding 'I recently gave up coffee so I am sleeping far better'. Whilst it's not necessary to give coffee up altogether, if you have problems sleeping, it's best not to drink it after 2 p.m. Alternatively, you could try drinking decaffeinated coffee.

Caffeine is a strong stimulant and the effects can last for hours. Research has shown that one cup of coffee at bedtime can lead to problems in getting to sleep and affect sleep quality – especially that of deep sleep. A cup of instant coffee contains on average 54 mg, whilst a cup of ground coffee averages 105 mg. A cup of tea averages 40 mg, so drinking it near bedtime is also inadvisable if you have trouble dropping off. Another option is Redbush tea, which is caffeine-free.

A glass of cola contains between 25 mg and 100 mg of caffeine. Cocoa isn't quite as bad – a cup contains, on average, just 5 mg. Remember, chocolate also contains caffeine – plain chocolate contains the most. According to the Food Standards Agency, a 50 g bar of plain chocolate contains up to 50 mg, whilst milk chocolate contains about half of that amount. The National Sleep Foundation website (see Directory) offers a caffeine calculator and caffeine counter card to help you work out how much caffeine you consume.

No nicotine

As well as being extremely damaging to your health in general, nicotine is also a stimulant, so if you must smoke, avoid smoking at bedtime. If you're using nicotine patches to help you stop smoking, be warned that they may cause vivid nightmares!

37. Try sleep-promoting supplements

This section covers the various herbal and other supplements that are reported to promote restful sleep. Generally, if you don't notice an improvement in your symptoms within three months of taking them, it's unlikely you will, so it may then be advisable to discontinue the treatment. It's wise to be wary of claims of a miraculous cure – sceptics point out there's little solid scientific evidence that supplements aid sleep, but there is plenty of anecdotal evidence. At the very least, a combination of these herbs could help you to unwind at the end of a busy day. Remember that herbal remedies are medicines, and like any medicine, they may have adverse effects. They may also interact with other medications. Always inform your GP if you are taking herbal medicines or other supplements.

Some over-the-counter products are unregistered. This means there's no guarantee of their content and quality. Once EU legislation has come into force in April 2011, safety levels should improve. In the meantime, make sure you buy products from a reputable company – if in doubt, always ask your GP or pharmacist. The Medicines and Healthcare Products Regulatory Agency (MHRA) offers further advice and information about using herbal medicines safely. The contact details are in the Directory.

Melatonin

Melatonin is a hormone that's made in the brain by converting tryptophan to serotonin and then to melatonin. It is secreted at night by the pineal gland in the brain to induce and maintain sleep. Melatonin supplements are widely used as sleep aids, but there's little scientific evidence that melatonin improves sleep patterns. In the UK melatonin is used as a short-term treatment for insomnia and is only available on prescription from a GP, under the brand name Circadin. Newspaper journalist and chronic insomniac Jessica Bown recently reported that when she was prescribed melatonin for a year it helped her to drift off more easily whilst she worked on changing her behaviour and attitude to sleep.

5HTP (5-hydroxytryptophan)

5HTP (5-hydroxytryptophan), usually derived from the West African Griffonia plant, is the precursor to serotonin, hence its promotion as a sleep aid. Several double-blind studies (where some participants are given a treatment and others are given a placebo, but neither the participants or the researchers are aware of who has received which) have suggested that 5HTP supplementation helps people to fall asleep quicker and stay asleep for longer. It's also thought to increase the amount of deep and REM sleep. The recommended dosage is 100 mg at bedtime. 5HTP shouldn't be taken alongside anti-depressants such as Prozac, as it may interact negatively with them.

St John's wort

St John's wort is well known for its antidepressant qualities. It's also an aid to sleep, especially where insomnia is linked to depression. It's thought to help regulate levels of serotonin and melatonin. St John's wort can react with some prescribed drugs so if you think you might be affected, speak to your GP or pharmacist before using it.

Hops

The flowers from hops are a popular herbal sleeping aid. They're thought to have tranquilising properties and are especially recommended for insomnia linked to anxiety and stress. Herbalists advise against using hops if you suffer from depression.

Valerian

Research has suggested that valerian, sometimes known as 'nature's valium', can help to reduce anxiety and promote sound sleep. Professor Jim Horne said recently that the herb appears to be 'the most effective of all herbal treatments for insomnia'. Smokers in particular seem to benefit from its effects. Valerian contains GABA (gamma-aminobutyric acid), an amino acid which is thought to help regulate sleep. Herbalists recommend taking valerian for four to six weeks and then taking a two to three week break.

Passion flower

Passion flower is a traditional South American remedy for insomnia. It has a mild sedative effect and is especially recommended for people who have trouble staying asleep. It's most effective when it's combined with other sleep-inducing herbs, so it's often found in proprietary preparations (see below).

Skullcap

It's claimed that skullcap relieves nervous tension, depression, pain and muscle cramps and also has a sedative effect, making it useful for insomnia. Native to the US, it was listed as a tranquilliser in the US Pharmacopoeia in 1863.

Vervain

The old English name for vervain was holy wort and it was one of the druids' seven sacred herbs. It has sedative and relaxing properties and has been traditionally used for insomnia and depression.

Wild Lettuce

Wild lettuce is thought to have pain-relieving, mild sedative and hypnotic properties and has been used to treat sleep disorders since Roman times.

Note:

There are various herbal products you can buy to help induce sleep, containing different combinations of these herbs. These include Gerard House Somnus Sleep, Kalms Sleep, Nytol Herbal, Sleep Herbal Tonic and Potter's Femmeherb Sweet Dreams. For more details, see Useful Products.

Chapter 6

Sleep Disorders

It's estimated that around only three per cent of the population suffer from medically recognised sleep disorders, including chronic insomnia. Apart from insomnia, there are over 70 different classifications of sleep disorders – most of which fall under these categories:

Sleep-related breathing disorders – e.g. snoring and sleep apnoeas
Sleep-related movement disorders – e.g. restless legs syndrome (RLS)
Circadian rhythm disorders – e.g. advanced sleep phase syndrome (ASPS) and delayed sleep phase syndrome (DSPS)
Parasomnias – e.g. sleepwalking
Hypersomnias – e.g. narcolepsy

38. Find out whether you have a sleep disorder

Specific sleep disorders can be linked to poor sleep and daytime sleepiness. It's important to be aware of the most common ones, so that you can determine whether or not they are at the root of your sleep problems. Once these have been ruled out or treated, you can focus on identifying the aspects of your lifestyle and behaviour that may be affecting your sleep. The London Sleep Centre offers a useful online sleep assessment tool to help you to find out whether you have a sleep disorder – see the Directory.

Sleep-related breathing disorders

This is a group of breathing disorders that can affect breathing patterns during sleep. Snoring and sleep apnoea are the most common types.

Snoring

It's thought that around 40 per cent of adults in the UK snore and over 30 million people (presumably some of the snorers as well their partners/families) suffer disrupted sleep as a result. Snoring is a sleep-related breathing disorder that can be triggered by being overweight, drinking alcohol at bedtime, taking sleeping pills, smoking and sleep apnoea (see below). Snoring is defined as loud upper-airway breathing caused by the tissues behind the nose and mouth vibrating. It happens when the airways are partially closed, because of a lack of muscle tone in the neck. This leads to air turbulence and the resulting noise.

Snoring can't be cured, but it can be controlled through lifestyle changes such as losing weight, stopping smoking and not drinking alcohol at bedtime. Other effective measures include sleeping on your side and sleeping on a firmer, thicker pillow to raise your head. There are also various anti-snoring products available, such as nasal strips and sprays. The British Snoring and Apnoea Association (see Directory) offers simple tests to identify the cause(s) of snoring, as well anti-snoring advice, tips and products. If your partner's or a family member's snoring is disupting your sleep, you will obviously want them to seek a solution. Perhaps the main hurdle is convincing them that they do snore! Taping or videoing the snorer can provide the proof and the motivation to do something about it. If your snoring, or someone else's, continues to disrupt your sleep, you or they need to seek medical advice.

Obstructive sleep apnoea

The term apnoea means 'without breath'. Sleep apnoea is a condition where the sufferer doesn't breathe properly during sleep and is the most common form of sleep-related breathing disorder. Obstructive sleep apnoea is the most common type and happens when the muscles controlling the upper airway relax during sleep. If they relax too much, the upper airway narrows, leading to snoring in some people and breathing problems if the airway becomes too narrow. Sometimes the airway becomes totally blocked and the person stops breathing temporarily, causing the sufferer to wake up to breathe before going back to sleep. This can last for ten seconds or more and can happen as many as 400 times during the night, leaving the sufferer exhausted the following day. Often the sufferer can't even remember waking up. The condition is often caused by reduced muscle tone or excess fat in the neck. Most people with sleep apnoea snore, but not everyone who snores has the condition. It's thought to affect all age groups and both sexes; however, it's most common in middle-aged men. Around one in 25 middle-aged men have the condition, compared to one in 50 middle-aged women in the UK.

The main symptoms of sleep apnoea are extreme tiredness and a tendency to fall asleep during the daytime. Always see your GP if you suspect you have the condition, as research suggests that it can put a strain on the cardiovascular system, increasing the risk of high blood pressure, heart disease and stroke. Sleeping on your side, losing weight and cutting out alcohol and smoking can be enough to relieve the symptoms. Otherwise, depending on the severity of the sleep apnoea, medication, a continuous positive air pressure device (CPAP) or surgery may be offered. Both The Sleep Apnoea Trust Association and The British Snoring and Sleep Apnoea Association offer information and advice on the condition (see Directory).

Sleep-related movement disorders

There are four main forms of sleep-related movement disorder: periodic limb movement disorder, restless legs syndrome, sleep bruxism (teeth grinding) and sleep-related rhythmic movement disorder.

Periodic limb movement disorder (PLMD)

PLMD is a sleep disorder where the sufferer repeatedly makes kicking and jerking movements with their legs during sleep, often without being aware of it. The movements disturb the sufferer's sleep and usually their partner's, so there's often daytime sleepiness. The condition is often linked to sleep apnoea and narcolepsy. Women are more likely to suffer from the condition than men. Other causes include too much caffeine, stress and mental health problems. Treatments for PLMD include benzodiazepines such as Clonazepam, or opioids such as codeine or methadone.

Restless legs syndrome (RLS)

RLS is a type of sleep-related movement disorder where you have an irresistible urge to move your legs. Sufferers may feel sensations of pain, tingling, itching or prickling which are relieved by moving the legs, but return as soon as the legs are still again, making sleep difficult. The syndrome can be caused by iron deficiency anaemia or folic acid deficiency and there may be a genetic link for some types. Some pregnant women suffer from the condition – especially in the last trimester of pregnancy. The symptoms may also be due to another underlying condition such as diabetes, rheumatoid arthritis, neurological diseases or Parkinson's disease. Certain drugs can make RLS worse – these include antidepressants, calcium blockers, anti-nausea medications (not domperidone), some anti-allergy drugs and too much caffeine. RLS may be helped by ensuring your diet contains adequate amounts of iron, folic acid and minerals such as calcium, potassium and magnesium (see Chapter 5 – Snooze Foods and Supplements). Walking, stretching and yoga may also help to relieve the symptoms.

Sleep bruxism

Teeth grinding or clenching (sleep bruxism) affects about 8 per cent of people and disrupts the sleep of both the sufferer and their bed partner. The condition is most common in people with sleep apnoea, heavy drinkers, smokers and coffee drinkers. It's also linked to anxiety, stress and dental problems. It's fairly common in children, who tend to 'grow out of it'. Not surprisingly, the teeth grinding can cause headaches, muscle aches and damage to the teeth. The condition can be treated with a combination of stress management techniques, lifestyle changes – such as cutting down on alcohol and coffee and stopping smoking – and with the use of a plastic splint or tooth guard during the night.

Sleep-related rhythmic movement disorder

This takes the form of banging the head or rocking the body and is most common in babies and young children. In older children it's linked to attention deficit hyperactivity disorder and happens during light sleep. In adults it can take place during any of the sleep stages. Treatment may include sleep restriction therapy and sleeping pills.

Circadian rhythm disorders

Circadian rhythm disorders are due to irregularities of the biological (body) clock. There are two main types of sleep/wake cycle disorders:

primary, where your biological clock is running at a different time to normal; and secondary, where your biological clock has been affected by a change in your waking and sleeping patterns, e.g. through shift work or long distance travel. The main symptom is insomnia or extreme daytime sleepiness.

There are two main forms – advanced sleep phase syndrome (ASPS) and delayed sleep phase syndrome (DSPS). ASPS is really an extreme version of the 'lark' sleeping pattern, where the sufferer can't stay awake in the evening and wakes very early in the morning, whereas DSPS is like an exaggerated version of an 'owl's' sleep pattern. Both types of disorder can be corrected by gradually rescheduling sleep patterns until they become more 'normal'. Exposure to bright light in the morning can help a DSPS sufferer to sleep earlier and exposure to bright light in the evening can help an ASPS sufferer to stay up later. Melatonin supplements, which are only available on subscription (see Chapter 5 – Snooze Foods and Supplements), can also help to regulate the sleep/wake cycle.

Night cramps

Night cramps are actually leg cramps that happen during the night, often disrupting sleep. The pain is caused by a leg muscle contracting too tightly. The affected muscles are usually one of the calf muscles behind and below the knee, or occasionally the muscles in the feet. One theory as to why they happen during sleep is that the muscles are already shortened when the knees are slightly bent in the natural sleep position. As you turn over during sleep the muscle contracts still further, leading to cramp. Other causes include dehydration, diabetes, hormonal fluctuations and B vitamin, magnesium, calcium and potassium deficiencies. Diuretics (including tea, coffee and alcohol) and some medications can also trigger them.

First and foremost, make sure you are eating a balanced diet that provides a wide range of vitamins and minerals (see Chapter 5 – Snooze Foods and Supplements). There are other steps you can take to help prevent cramps. Gently stretching your calf muscles before bedtime can help. Yoga postures are particularly good for this. Massaging your calves before bedtime may relax the muscles. There's also an over-the-counter medicine called Crampex that contains calcium and niacin (vitamin B3). The product manufacturer provides a website with useful tips and information, including leg stretching exercises to help prevent cramps (see Useful Products). Quinine tablets are commonly prescribed for night cramps.

Parasomnias

Parasomnias are a group of sleep disorders that involve movement during sleep, or seeing, hearing or feeling things that aren't there. They include sleepwalking and nightmares. The well-loved actress Julie Walters recently wrote in her autobiography of how she had suffered from disturbed sleep, punctuated by nightmares and sleepwalking, since childhood. She found that hypnotherapy in her late forties helped to dispel her night terrors and sleepwalking, and then a few years later acupuncture helped her sleep more soundly.

Sleepwalking

In 2007 Travelodge's 'Director of Sleep', Leigh McCarron, reported that the company's staff had dealt with over 400 cases of sleepwalking in the past year, suggesting that sleepwalking was on the rise. The sleepwalkers were mainly men and most appeared at reception attempting to check out, or buy a newspaper!

Sleepwalking is a general term used to describe disorders where people perform activities during their sleep and can include simple movements like sitting up and looking around or walking around and performing tasks normally done whilst awake. The most common type of sleepwalking is called somnambulism, which is most prevalent in children, but also affects about one or two per cent of adults. Sleepwalking happens during deep sleep and there's a strong genetic link. It's often linked to over-tiredness, stress, sleeping pills, alcohol – anything that can prevent the brain from awakening easily. Often the trigger is needing to go to the toilet. Sleep apnoeas and periodic limb movements can also be involved. Adopting a regular bedtime and ensuring you don't become over-tired are effective preventative measures, but if it persists, you should seek specialist help.

Nightmares

Nightmares are a common form of parasomnia. There are two main types: idiopathic, where the cause isn't known and post-traumatic, where the nightmares are experienced after a distressing event and may involve re-living it.

The main difference between a bad dream and a nightmare is that the latter will wake you up. The images tend to be vivid and the plots are often complex, involving disturbing feelings, which seem to stem from fear, anxiety, grief and anger. There seems to be a genetic link, and many people who have nightmares during childhood tend to continue to have them during adulthood. Stress management and relaxation techniques may help nightmares where there is no obvious cause, whilst counselling or at least talking things through with a trustworthy person may help to reduce nightmares linked to a traumatic event.

Hypersomnias

Hypersomnias involve a person getting too much or too little sleep, or being unable to control their patterns of sleep or sleepiness and include menstrual-related hypersomnia and hypersomnia due to a medical condition.

Narcolepsy

The best known of this group of conditions is narcolepsy. It's estimated to affect around one in two thousand people, though it may be under-reported. It's thought to be caused by the faulty control of the sleep/wake cycle and REM sleep in particular. The main symptoms are insomnia, excessive daytime sleepiness and uncontrollable sleep attacks. Other symptoms include:

- Temporary paralysis when falling asleep or waking up
- Hallucinations involving vivid images or sounds on falling asleep or awakening.
- Moments or longer periods of trance-like behaviour, where everyday activities are carried out on autopilot so that afterwards the sufferer can't remember doing them
- Waking up frequently during the night, feeling alert and agitated
- There may also be flushes and a rapid heartbeat

The condition can start before the age of 15, but usually begins between the ages of 20 and 40. It's thought to be linked to a lack of orexin, a brain chemical that promotes alertness. Treatment includes stimulant drugs, such as Modafinil, as well as lifestyle changes and coping strategies. The Narcolepsy Association UK (UKAN) offers more information and advice on the condition – see the Directory.

Chapter 7

Sleep Medications

There was a time when sleeping pills were commonly prescribed for insomnia. Today doctors are more aware of the problems they can cause and their limited ability to improve sleep, so they are less likely to prescribe them. This chapter considers when sleeping pills may be helpful and looks at some of the over-the-counter and prescribed drugs commonly recommended for insomnia and their possible side effects.

39. Consider sleeping pills as a short-term solution

In the long term, if you follow the various psychological and behavioural approaches outlined in this book, you are likely to notice big improvements in your sleep patterns. But if you suffer from chronic insomnia, or particularly severe acute insomnia and need a temporary reprieve to help you cope until your lifestyle changes begin to have an effect, you may want to try over-the-counter or prescription sleeping pills.

In the short term, sleeping pills can be a useful crutch, but they don't offer a long-term solution. They don't treat the causes of your insomnia – they merely mask the symptoms. Nor do they encourage a deep, restful sleep – they tend to increase stage two light sleep and reduce stage four deep sleep and REM sleep. According to Professor Jim Horne, after a few weeks of taking sleeping tablets, most users will gain no more than 20 minutes sleep and few will find the time taken to fall asleep reduced by more than 15 minutes. The NHS recommends that GPs prescribe short courses, to avoid dependency.

The singer and actress Toyah Wilcox knows only too well about the problems that can arise from taking prescription sleeping pills. She told recently of how, having suffered from insomnia since the age of 14, she was prescribed temazepam at the age of 25. For the first time in years she enjoyed eight hours' sleep each night, but she soon found herself unable to sleep without sleeping pills and eventually noticed they were less effective, as she developed a tolerance to them. After a couple of years she decided she didn't want to be 'controlled by pills', so she stopped taking them, saying 'never again'. She still considers four hours to be a good night's sleep. Perhaps her attitude to sleep is at the root of her problem – she admits to viewing it as 'boring' and 'a waste of time'.

Julie Walters had a similar experience when she began taking sleeping pills for her insomnia – at the time she was rehearsing for the the musical version of *Acorn Antiques* and was exhausted from lack of sleep. Her husband suggested she should try sleeping tablets, which she did, explaining, 'They helped for a while, but of course they don't after a time and then you have to keep building up the dose, and you can't do that.'

So the main message is that sleeping pills should only be viewed as a short-term solution to help you re-establish more normal sleep patterns.

40. Find out more about over-the-counter sleeping pills

These are usually antihistamines, such as dipenhydramine and promethazine, which were originally used to treat allergies, but once they were found to cause daytime drowsiness they were redeveloped as over-the-counter medications to help insomnia. They don't work as well as prescription drugs, but could be viewed as the next step if herbal remedies and supplements haven't helped. They shouldn't be taken with alcohol and can cause grogginess the next day if taken too late at night. Other possible side effects include a dry mouth, blurred vision and stomach upsets. As is the case with sleeping pills, you can develop a tolerance, which means you need to keep increasing the dose to get the same results. Products containing dipenhydramine include Nytol, which is promoted as a treatment for temporary sleeplessness due to factors such as stress, or jet lag. Only one box can be bought at a time, as this medication shouldn't be taken for longer than two weeks without seeing your GP. Dreemon is another similar product. Over-the-counter products containing promethazine include Phenergan and Sominex.

Note:

Over-the-counter sleeping pills shouldn't be taken by anyone with angina, glaucoma, or prostrate or urinary problems, nor alongside anti-nausea or travel-sickness medications. If in doubt, always speak to your pharmacist or GP first.

41. Give your GP helpful information

Before prescribing sleeping pills, or any other form of treatment, your GP will need to know as much as possible about your sleep problem – this is where keeping a sleep diary can be useful (see Introduction). If you haven't kept a diary, note down the answers to these questions as accurately as you can before you go to your appointment:

- Do you find it difficult to fall asleep?
- Roughly how long does it take you to drop off?
- Do you wake frequently during the night?
- Do you wake up too early in the morning?
- Do you feel anxious or depressed?
- How long have you had a sleep problem for?
- Do you feel tired during the day?
- Do you function efficiently during the day?

42. Learn about prescription sleeping pills

Benzodiazepines

These include temazepam, nitrazepam, lormetazepam and diazepam. They are used to calm you down and make you feel sleepy and are especially useful if anxiety is causing insomnia. But the downside is tolerance – as your body gets used to the drug, higher doses are needed to get the same effects. Other problems include dependency, which means you end up only being able to sleep when you take the pills, and rebound, which is where symptoms worsen when you stop taking them. Common side effects include drowsiness or dizziness the following day. Recent research has linked these effects to an increased risk of being involved in a road accident. Benzodiazepines shouldn't be taken with alcohol, because they enhance its effects.

'Z' drugs

These include the hypnotic medications zolpidem, zopiclone and zaleplon. They help to promote sleep in most cases and seem to cause fewer side effects than benzodiazepines, though there still may be problems with dependence and withdrawal. Plus, like benzodiazepines, there's evidence of an increased risk of being involved in a road accident the day after using them. They are also more expensive than benzodiazepines; the UK's National Institute of Clinical Excellence (NICE) ruled that, as there is no firm evidence of differences in the effects of these drugs, doctors should work out the costs for each patient and prescribe the cheapest.

Antidepressants

These include amitriptyline, dothiepin, clonazepam, venlafaxine, mirtazapine and trazadone. These are usually given in low doses and act as sedatives. Evidence suggests they can help where insomnia is linked to depression. Common side effects include a dry mouth and blurred vision and there may be difficulty in urinating, sweating and an irregular heartbeat. Withdrawal from antidepressants needs to be gradual, to avoid a rebound effect.

Chapter 8

DIY Complementary Therapies

Complementary therapies seek to treat the whole person, rather than just the symptoms. The emphasis is on supporting the body to enable it to heal itself. Whilst it's unlikely any complementary treatment will 'cure' your insomnia, some may help you to relax and improve your general well-being – which may in turn help to promote sound sleep.

Experts from the medical profession are beginning to accept that complementary therapies may have a place in the tratment of insomnia. Doctor Philip S. Eichling, from the Sleep Disorders Centre at the University of Arizona College of Medicine, recently concluded that 'the most promising use of complementary and alternative medicine (CAM) is in the area of insomnia'. He pointed out that meditation, stress management, relaxation therapies and massage all fitted easily into the behaviour change and relaxation therapies currently used in sleep medicine. He added that although acupuncture and 'energy therapies' – e.g. reflexology and acupressure – hadn't been adequately studied, 'given the mind/body nature of insomnia, positive outcomes wouldn't be surprising'.

This chapter provides an overview and evaluation of complementary therapies that could help insomnia and suggests techniques and treatments you can try for yourself at home.

43. Apply acupressure

Acupressure is part of traditional Chinese medicine and is often described as 'acupuncture without needles'. Like acupuncture, it's based on the idea that life energy, or qi, flows through channels in the body known as meridians. An even passage of qi throughout the body is viewed as vital to good health. Disruption of the flow of qi in a meridian can lead to illness at any point along it. The flow of qi can be affected by various factors, including stress, emotional distress, diet and environment. Qi is the most concentrated at points along the meridians known as acupoints. There's scientific evidence that stimulating particular acupoints can relieve both pain and nausea. However, evidence that suggests acupuncture and related treatments (including acupressure) can help insomnia was recently reviewed: the conclusion was that though they *may* improve sleep quality, further, more rigorous testing was needed to prove this.

You can try the following simple acupressure techniques for yourself:

'Third eye'

To help induce sleep, use the middle finger of your left hand to gently massage the 'third eye' point, which is situated in between the eyebrows.

'Close eyes'

To work the Ki 6 or 'close eyes' acupoint, use your right thumb to massage the inside of the left heel gently in a circular motion, then apply pressure for a few seconds. Repeat on the right heel, using the left thumb.

'Calm sleep'

To work the Bl 62 or 'calm sleep' acupoint, follow the instructions for the 'close eyes' acupoint, only massage the *outside* of the heels.

44. Sleep easy with essential oils

Essential oils are extracted from the roots, stalks, leaves and flowers of plants. Aromatherapy is based on the theory that scents released from essential oils affect the hypothalamus, the part of the brain which controls the glands and hormonal system, thus influencing mood and lowering stress levels. When used in massage, baths and compresses, the oils are absorbed into the bloodstream and transported to the organs and glands, which benefit from their healing effects.

Because of their effects on the mind and emotions, essential oils have long been used to help induce sleep. Inhaling lavender oil at night has been shown to be as effective as commonly prescribed sleeping tablets for treating insomnia, helping to improve sleep quality by 20 per cent. To benefit from its calming, soothing, sedative properties, try sprinkling a few drops of neat oil on your pillow at night. Using lavender oil during the day could also help to improve sleep by aiding stress management. Japanese researchers recently reported that sniffing lavender oil for five minutes daily dramatically reduces the stress hormone cortisol. Rosemary oil was found to be equally effective at reducing stress.

Alternatively, add six drops of lavender oil to a warm bedtime bath, or use it for massage, diluted in a carrier oil such as almond, grapeseed or olive oil.

Clary sage can be used in the same way, but it's a strong relaxant, so don't combine it with alcohol, as it may cause nightmares!

If a stuffy nose from cold or flu causes sleep problems, sprinkle a few drops of tea tree or eucalptus oil on your pillow.

In her book, *Aromatherapy: An A–Z*, aromatherapist Patricia Davis also recommends camomile and neroli essential oils, saying she has found these two oils, along with lavender, 'the most effective in helping insomnia'. She suggests varying the oils you use if you need help with sleeping for more than a week or two.

45. Feng shui your bedroom

Feng shui means 'wind and water' and is the ancient Chinese art of creating a balanced, harmonius environment to promote health, wealth and happiness. It involves ensuring that the layout of a building, and everything in it, allows the free flow of energy or *chi*. Another main feature of feng shui is ensuring there is balance between *yin* (female, passive) and *yang* (male, active) energies. Practitioners claim that a building can affect the behaviour, emotions, thoughts and health of the people who spend time in it.

Follow these feng shui tips for a restful sleep:

- Remove clutter to encourage the flow of *chi* – get rid of clothes and shoes that you don't wear.
- Don't store things under the bed where they can block *chi* and disrupt sleep.
- Don't keep items on top of the wardrobe. Keep your dressing table tidy and only display items you use regularly.

- Place your bed as far away from the bedroom door as possible, with the headboard against a solid wall and in a position where you can see the door, so that you feel supported and safe.

- Choose a wooden-framed bed with a solid headboard to protect your *chi* whilst you sleep.

- Choose paints and soft furnishings in pale blue or violet – *yin* shades that promote serenity and calm.

- Lighting needs to be more *yin* than usual to promote relaxation and sleep, so use dimmer switches, bedside lamps with rounded shades and candles.

- Avoid keeping electrical equipment, such as a television or computer, in your bedroom as they produce too much *yang* energy. Use a battery-operated alarm clock rather than an electrical one.

- Don't position a mirror so that it reflects the bed, as this may disrupt sleep.

46. Use flower power

Flower essences have been used for their healing properties for thousands of years. However, it was Dr Edward Bach, a Harley Street doctor, bacteriologist and homeopath, who developed their use in the twentieth century. Bach identified 38 basic negative states of mind and devised a plant or flower based remedy for each. The remedies are thought to help counteract negative emotions, such as despair, fear and uncertainty, but there's only anecdotal evidence regarding their effectiveness. They're widely available in pharmacies in easy-to-carry 10- and 20-ml phials.

Bach's Rescue Remedy is designed to help you cope with times of acute stress and may help with related sleep problems. White chestnut is recommended where unwanted thoughts and worries prevent you from sleeping. Mimulus for fear, or rock rose for terror, may help where nightmares disturb sleep. The remedies can usually be taken by diluting two drops in a glass of water and sipping at intervals. Alternatively, you can apply them directly to your skin, by rubbing them onto your lips, behind your ears or on your temples and wrists.

For further information to help you choose a suitable flower remedy and an online questionnaire that enables you to select a personalised blend, visit www.bachremedies.co.uk.

47. Get help from homeopathy

Homeopathy literally means 'same suffering' and is based on the idea that 'like cures like' – substances that can invoke symptoms in a well person can treat the same symptoms in a person who is ill. For example, coffee contains caffeine – excessive amounts are linked to an overactive mind and insomnia, so the remedy Coffea is often prescribed for these very symptoms (see list of remedies below).

Symptoms like inflammation or fever are viewed as an indication that the body is trying to heal itself. The theory is that homeopathic remedies encourage this self-healing process and that they work in a similar way to vaccines. Homeopaths warn that there can be a worsening of symptoms at first and that this signals that the body's healing mechanism has been stimulated.

The substances used in homeopathic remedies come from plant, animal, mineral, bark and metal sources. These substances are turned into a tincture, which is then diluted many times over. Homeopaths claim that the more diluted a remedy is, the higher its potency and the lower its potential side effects. They believe in the 'memory of water', the theory that even though the molecules from a substance have been diluted away, they've left behind an electromagnetic 'footprint' – rather like a recording on an audiotape – which still has an effect on the body.

These ideas are controversial and many GPs remain sceptical. Evidence to support homeopathy exists, but critics argue that much of it is inconclusive. For example, research published in 2005 reported improvements in symptoms and well-being among 70 per cent of patients receiving individualised homeopathy. The study involved 6,500 patients over a six-year period at the Bristol Homeopathic Hospital. Critics of the studies argue there was no comparison group and patients may have given a positive response because it was expected. However, many people claim to have been helped by homeopathy, so it may well be worth trying.

There are two main types of remedies – whole person based and symptom based. A homeopath would prescribe a remedy aimed at you as a whole person, based on your personality, as well as the symptoms you experience.

Below is a list of homeopathic remedies, along with the insomnia-related physical and psychological symptoms and personality types for which they're indicated. To self-prescribe, simply choose the remedy whose indications most closely match your symptoms. The recommended dose for each remedy is 30 c (1:100 dilution carried out 30 times) for up to ten consecutive nights. Repeat the dose if you waken during the night and can't get back to sleep.

Aconite

Aconite is useful where sleeplessness is linked to restlessness, nervousness, vivid dreams and nightmares. It's helpful for excitable, anxious personalities. Symptoms tend to improve with fresh air and perspiration, and are worsened when the bedroom is too warm and with exposure to tobacco smoke or loud music.

Avena sativa (oats)

Avena Sativa is recommended for chronic insomnia that's linked to nervous exhaustion. It's especially indicated for nervous or elderly people, or for those whose insomnia has stemmed from illness.

Coffea (coffee)

Recommended where sleep is fitful and linked to restlessness and an overstimulated mind that simply won't switch off. This may be due to the use of too many stimulants, such as coffee and nicotine. It's suitable for overexcitable personalities and where symptoms are improved by warmth and made worse by taking sleeping pills, noise and the cold.

Ignatia (agnate)

Ignatia is recommended when the sufferer is apprehensive about going to bed, because of the fear of never being able to sleep again. It's suitable for people with emotional problems and rapid mood changes – especially women – perhaps following a bereavement, or the breakdown of a relationship. Deep breathing and eating improves symptoms. Coffee, tobacco and alcohol make the symptoms worse.

Nux vomica

Indicated where insomnia is accompanied by irritability and nightmares. It's a good remedy for workaholic perfectionists who constantly push themselves. It's also useful where the insomnia is improved when lying on either side and with warmth, and made worse by lying on the back and eating too much – especially spicy foods – coldness and noise.

You can also buy products containing a combination of these remedies, such as Nelsons Noctura (see Useful Products).

48. Relax with reflexology

Reflexology is based on the idea that the body has ten energy zones that run vertically from the feet and hands up to the head. Reflexologists believe that a blockage in the flow of energy along one of these zones will affect the functioning of the organs, glands, bones and muscles that lie within it, and lead to illness. These blockages manifest themselves as granular deposits in the relevant reflex, causing tenderness. Corns, bunions and even hard skin are thought to indicate problems in the parts of the body their position relates to. The energy theory behind reflexology is very similar to the one underpinning acupressure, though practitioners claim it's a different system.

It is claimed that stimulating the reflexes with the fingers and thumbs breaks down the granular deposits, releasing the flow of energy and and encouraging self-healing in the affected parts of the body.

A recent small study at the University of Ulster suggested that reflexology can help those suffering from insomnia to sleep better.

Hand-y relaxer

To relieve stress and tension before bedtime, apply pressure to the solar plexuses. Place your left hand, palm facing upwards, in your right hand, with your right thumb uppermost. Locate the area about two-thirds of the way up your left palm, in line with the centre of your middle finger, then press down firmly with your right thumb using a clockwise rotational movement. Repeat on the right hand using the left thumb.

Cycle balancer

To help balance your sleep/wake cycle, try this DIY reflexology technique. It stimulates your pineal gland, which produces the sleep hormone melatonin. Using your thumb and forefinger, apply pressure to the fleshy area about two-thirds of the way up each of your big toes for a couple of minutes. Do this an hour or so before bedtime.

49. Massage away stress

Massage is one of the oldest and most effective methods of counteracting stress. Daily tensions and stress can make us tense and lead to pain and muscle stiffness. The Greek philosopher Hippocrates – the 'father of medicine' – recognised the value of massage, claiming it 'can loosen a joint that is too rigid'. Massage involves touch – a powerful tool which can ease away tensions, aches and pains. It works by stimulating the release of endorphins – the body's own painkillers – and serotonin, which is associated with relaxation. It also decreases the level of stress hormones in the blood and improves blood circulation. Several studies have shown that babies sleep more soundly after a massage. One study reported that cancer patients experienced less pain and a better quality of sleep when they received a weekly massage. Another showed that massage benefitted sufferers of fibromyalgia (a condition leading to muscular pain, stiffness and fatigue) – they suffered less pain and slept for longer.

Make your own massage oil by mixing a few drops of a suitable aromatherapy oil (see '44. Sleep easy with essential oils') into a carrier oil such as almond or grapeseed. The easiest way to enjoy the benefits of massage is for you and a partner to massage each other's back, neck and shoulders, using the basic techniques outlined below:

Stroking/effleurage – glide both hands over the skin in rhythmic fanning or circular movements.

Kneading – using alternate hands, squeeze and release flesh between your fingers and thumbs, as if you're kneading dough.

Friction – use your thumbs to apply even pressure or make small circles on either side of the spine.

Hacking – use the sides of both hands in a relaxed state to give short, sharp taps all over.

Playing some relaxing music at the same time can enhance the feelings of relaxation.

50. Wind down with yoga

Because yoga is a gentle form of exercise that aids relaxation by taking your mind off your worries, it's ideal for practising early in the evening to help you to wind down before bedtime. Yoga also strengthens the body and increases flexibility. The word yoga stems from the Sanskrit word *yuj*, meaning union. Yoga postures and breathing exercises are designed to unite the body, mind and soul. They can help to promote sound sleep by calming the mind, relieving stress and tension and relaxing the muscles, easing aches and pains.

Yoga relaxation, which involves lying on your back in the Corpse Pose and tensing and relaxing the muscles step by step, is recommended if you have problems falling asleep. The Shoulderstand, an inverted (upside-down) pose, is also recommended to encourage relaxation before bedtime.

The best way to learn yoga is to attend classes run by a qualified teacher. To find one near you, go to the British Wheel of Yoga's website – www.bwy.org.uk. Or, if you'd prefer to teach yourself at home, visit www.abc-of-yoga.com, a site that offers an animated step-by-step guide to performing the various postures. The following websites also offer information, guidance and yoga products: www.yoga-abode.com, www.yogahealthguide.com and www.yogaatwork.co.uk.

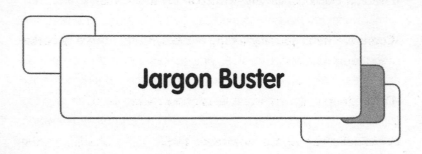

A glossary explaining the meaning of terms that may be used in connection with insomnia.

Actigraph – electronic device uses to measure brain activity and therefore sleep and wakefuless.

Advanced sleep phase syndrome (ASPS) – circadian rhythm disorder where the sufferer has problems staying awake in the evening and sleeping beyond the early hours.

Antihistamines – medicines usually used to treat allergies, some of which cause drowsiness, making them useful as a sleep aid.

Benzodiazepines – the group of drugs used to treat anxiety and sleep problems.

Cataplexy – muscle weakness found in narcolepsy sufferers.

Chronic insomnia – insomnia that lasts for longer than a month.

Circadian rhythm – internal body clock that controls the sleep/wake cycle.

Circadian rhythm disorders – disorders of the body clock that affect an individual's ability to sleep at the usual times.

Cognitive behavioural therapy – treatment that targets behaviour and thought processes.

Deep sleep – also known as delta or slow-wave sleep.

Delayed sleep phase syndrome (DSPS) – a circadian rhythm disorder where the body clock is running late. This leads to the sufferer finding it difficult to fall asleep until very late and having trouble getting up early.

Diuretic – a substance that promotes urination.

Double-blind – a trial in which information which may influence the behaviour of the investigators or the participants (such as which participants have been given a placebo rather than an active treatment) is withheld.

Drowsiness – the first stage of sleep, when your brainwaves begin to slow down.

Epworth sleepiness scale – scale devised to measure sleepiness during daytime activities.

Gamma-aminobutyric acid (GABA) – an amino acid that acts as a chemical messenger in the brain, spinal cord, heart, lungs and kidneys, and 'tells' the body to slow down.

Glycaemic index (GI) – a ranking of foods according to the effect they have on blood sugar levels.

Hypersomnias – sleep disorders involving excessive daytime sleep.

Insomnia – difficulty in falling or staying asleep.

Jet lag – temporary disruption of the body's sleep/wake cycle through air travel across different time zones.

Light sleep – the second stage of sleep.

Melatonin – a hormone produced in the pineal gland that promotes sleep.

Narcolepsy – a sleep disorder linked to excessive daytime sleepiness and insomnia.

Non-rapid eye movement (NREM) – the type of sleep that occurs during sleep stages one to four. It differs from stage five, rapid eye movement (REM), sleep in that there are no darting eye movements.

Parasomnias – sleep disorders involving movement, or seeing, hearing or feeling things that don't exist.

Periodic limb movement disorder – sleep disorder where sufferer moves limbs involuntarily whilst asleep.

Placebo – an inactive substance given to a patient to compare its effects with those of a treatment, or so that participants can benefit from believing they have received a treatment and will therefore feel better.

Rapid eye movement (REM) – the type of sleep that occurs during sleep stage five when the brain is most active and involves the eyes moving quickly whilst the eyelids are closed.

Restless legs syndrome (RLS) – a periodic limb movement disorder where the sufferer repeatedly moves the legs during sleep.

Serotonin – a substance the body uses to make the 'sleep hormone' melatonin. Also known as 5HT.

Short-term insomnia – insomnia that lasts up to one month.

Somnambulism – medical term for sleepwalking (one of the parasomnias).

Sleep apnoea – condition where sufferer momentarily stops breathing during sleep.

Sleep bruxism – teeth grinding at night.

Sleep homeostat – mechanism controlled by brain chemicals such as melatonin, that ensures you get enough sleep.

Sleep-onset insomnia – difficulty in falling asleep.

Sleep-maintenance insomnia – difficulty in staying asleep.

Sleep-related breathing disorders – sleep disorders that affect breathing during sleep, such as sleep apnoea.

Sleep-related movement disorders – group of disorders where sufferer makes involuntary movements during sleep.

Sleep/wake cycle –pattern of sleep and wakefulness that is determined by the circadian rhythm and sleep homeostat.

Stimulus control therapy – a treatment that aims to help insomnia by encouraging the brain to link certain cues, e.g. the bedroom, with sleep.

Transient insomnia – insomnia that lasts for just a few nights.

Tryptophan – an amino acid used to make serotonin, which is turned into the 'sleep hormone' melatonin.

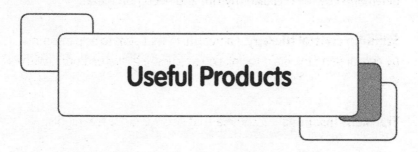

Useful Products

Below is a list of products that may help to ease insomnia. The author doesn't endorse or recommend any particular product and this list is by no means exhaustive.

Allersafe bedding

An anti-allergy product called Amicor Pure is woven into the bedding. This has both an anti-fungal and anti-bacterial effect which helps to keep dustmites at bay. The manufacturer claims that Allersafe bedding helps you to achieve a good night's sleep by managing the allergens which can lead to disturbed sleep patterns.
Telephone: 0800 1696685
Website: www.allersafe.co.uk

Asphalia for natural sleep

Supplement containing melatonin derived from a natural meadowgrass and white clover to help regulate sleep patterns.
Telephone: 0800 3898 195
Website: www.victoriahealth.com

Bach Rescue Night

A blend of flowers essences, including white chestnut, to help you 'switch off' and sleep soundly.

Telephone: 020 8773 3803
Website: www.bachshop.co.uk

Badger Sleep Balm
A balm containing pure essential oils of bergamot, ginger, rosemary, lavender and balsam fir to relax your mind and help send you to sleep.
Telephone: 0845 652 9591
Website: www.badgerbalm.bathandunwind.com

Better Sleep Pillow
An orthopaedic pillow with contours and support provided by memory foam. The manufacturer claims this product helps to prevent neck and shoulder pain and frozen shoulder, and promotes more restful sleep.
Website: www.bettersleeppillow.com

Boots Alternatives Sleep Well Cones
Adhesive acupressure point cones that gently massage the H7 (heart 7) point on the inside of the wrist to help promote natural sleep.
Website: www.boots.com

Chillow
A cooling pad that is activated by tap water. When placed on your pillow, it reduces your body temperature, helping induce sleep.
Telephone: 08700 117174
Website: www.chillow.co.uk

Clipper Organic Sleep Easy
Tea bags containing cinnamon, lemon balm, valerian root and chamomile to help you relax before bedtime.
Telephone (for stockists): 01308 863344
Website: www.clipper-teas.com

Crampex Tablets

Aim to help treat and prevent night muscle cramps. Contain calcium gluconate to help correct any calcium deficiency, cholecalciferol to aid calcium absorption and niacin to improve poor circulation.
Telephone: 01484 842217
Website: www.thorntonross.com/crampex

Earplugs

A wide range of foam, wax and silicone earplugs, ideal for blocking out unwanted noises when trying to sleep.
Telephone: 020 8861 3149
Website: www.snorestore.co.uk

Gerard House Somnus Sleep

A traditional herbal preparation containing hops, valerian and passion flower to relieve restlessness and promote relaxation and natural sleep.
Telephone: 0871 871 6611
Website: www.goodnessdirect.co.uk

HoMedics Sound Spa

A budget-priced portable sound machine that filters out background noise with six digitally recorded sounds: ocean, rain, rainforest, waterfall, heartbeat and summer night, with a self-timer for 15, 30 or 60 minutes.
Telephone: 08700 84 11 14
Website: www.auravita.com

Insomnia Relief Scent Inhaler

A blend of pure essential oils known to have calming effects, including lavender, chamomile and marjoram, to help promote sound sleep. Available from Victoria Health.

Telephone: 0800 3898 195
Website: www.victoriahealth.com

Kalms Sleep

Herbal supplement containing valerian, passion flower, wild lettuce vervain and hops. The manufacturer claims the product promotes sleep without leaving you feeling drowsy the next day.
Website: www.kalmssleep.com

Lavender Nights

A range of bath products that combine Bach flower remedies with pure organic English lavender and Melissa to help calm the body and mind.
Telephone: 020 8773 3803
Website: www.bachshop.co.uk

Lumie Bodyclock

A clock that helps to regulate the sleep/wake cycle by simulating sunrise to waken you gently and naturally. Options include a clock with white noise and one offering a guided sleep meditation.
Telephone: 01954 780 500
Website: www.lumie.com

Natural Sleep Inducement

A musical CD designed to help you drift off to sleep. Tracks include 'Blue Horizon', 'Eternal Wave' and 'Celestial Glow'.
Telephone: 0870 199 3260
Website: www.feelkarma.com

Nelsons Noctura

A combination of homeopathic remedies including Kali brom., Coffea, Passiflora and Avena sativa, aimed to relieve insomnia. Available from supermarkets and pharmacies nationwide.

Telephone: 020 7629 3118
Website: www.nelsonshomeopathy.co.uk

Nytol Herbal Tablets
A combination of hops, valerian and passion flower to help promote calmness and restful sleep.
Telephone: 020 8047 2700
Website: www.nytol.co.uk

Potter's Femmeherb Sweet Dreams
Herbal tablets containing passion flower extract, which is renowned for its sedative, calming qualities.
Telephone: 0871 871 6611
Website: www.goodnessdirect.co.uk

Sleep Earplugs
A wide range of foam, wax and silicone earplugs, ideal for blocking out unwanted noises when trying to sleep.
Telephone: 020 8861 3149
Website: www.snorestore.co.uk

Sleep Herbal Tonic
A drink containing lavender, valerian, chamomile flowers, skullcap, passion flower and lime blossom. Recommended for those having problems sleeping due to stress, 'mental chatter' or over-exhaustion, as well as those that wake during the night.
Telephone: 0800 3898 195
Website: www.victoriahealth.com

Sleep Soundly CD
A CD with either music or nature soundtracks, offering subliminal messages to help send you off to sleep. Play at night to hear

affirmations such as 'Sleep restores me. Sleep refreshes me. I sleep deeply. I sleep peacefully'.
Telephone: 01628 898366
Website: www.vitalia-health.co.uk

Sleep Well Mist
A spray containing lavender oil and flower essences to help reassure, relax and ease a worried mind.
Telephone: 0800 3898 195
Website: www.victoriahealth.com

Soothie Eye Mask
A sleep mask filled with linseeds and fragranced with lavender to help you relax.
Telephone: 01394 670970
Website: www.snoozeshop.com

Helpful Books

Davis, Adelle, *Let's Eat Right To Keep Fit* (Thorson's New Ed Edition, 1995) – this book was first published way back in 1954, yet its message – that eating a balanced diet is the cornerstone of good health – is as important as ever. The author clearly explains the functions of essential nutrients and identifies the best sources.

Espie, Colin A., *Overcoming Insomnia and Sleep Problems* (Robinson Publishing, 2006) – a detailed guide to using cognitive behavioural techniques to help you overcome insomnia and sleep problems, written by a leading member of the American Academy of Sleep Medicine and the British Sleep Society.

Idzikowski, Chris, Dr, *Sleep: The Secret to Sleeping Well and Waking Refreshed* (Collins, 2007) – a comprehensive guide to sleep and sleep disorders, written by the director of the Edinburgh Sleep Centre.

Kryger, Meir, Dr, *Can't Sleep, Can't Stay Awake: A Woman's Guide to Sleep Disorders* (US Adaptations, 2007) – an in-depth guide as to why women sleep differently to men and suffer from sleep problems more often.

Wiedman, John, *Desperately Seeking Snoozin': The Insomnia Cure From Awake to Zzzz* (University of Wisconsin Press, 1998) –this is a detailed account of how the author beat long-term insomnia by following a pre-sleep relaxation routine and restricting his time in bed.

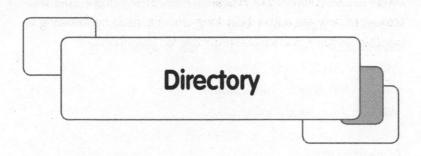

Directory

Below is a list of useful contacts that offer information and advice on insomnia and related topics.

American Academy of Sleep Medicine

America's leading professional organisation specialising in sleep medicine, education and research. Also publishes the journal Sleep in collaboration with the Sleep Research Society.

Website: www.aasmnet.org

American Insomnia Association

A patient-based organisation that is dedicated to assisting and providing resources to individuals who suffer from insomnia. The AIA advocates and promotes awareness, education and research of insomnia disorders. The website offers detailed information about insomnia.

Website: www.americaninsomniaassociation.org

BBC Science and Nature

Part of the BBC's website offering information on science and nature, including the human body.

Website: www.bbc.co.uk/sn

The British Snoring and Sleep Apnoea Association

A not-for-profit organisation dedicated to helping snorers and their bed partners improve their sleep.

Address: Castle Court, 41 London Road, Reigate, RH2 9RJ

Telephone: 01737 245638

E-mail: info@britishsnoring.co.uk

Website: www.britishsnoring.co.uk

Circadian.com

A US website offering shiftworkers advice on sleep, health, exercise and managing family life.

Website: www.circadian.com

Good Sleep Advice

A campaign supported by Crampex medication for night cramps. The website offers information and advice on how to sleep better.

Website: www.goodsleepadvice.com

Insomnia Helpline

Run by the Medical Advisory Service. Trained nurses are available to talk through your problems and, where necessary, refer you on to appropriate sources of help and advice.

Address: Medical Advisory Service, PO Box 3087, London, W4 4ZP

Telephone: 020 8994 9874

Email: info@medicaladvisoryservice.org.uk

Website: www.medicaladvisoryservice.org.uk

Insomniacs.co.uk

A website formed to offer a unique reference point on how to overcome insomnia, sleeping problems and sleep disorders. The site

contains features and articles written by journalists and experts with a particular interest, or background, in insomnia. You can also sign up for a free monthly newsletter.
Website: www.insomniacs.co.uk

The Laughter Network

A group of professionals whose aim is to bring more happiness and laughter into people's lives. Provides information about the health benefits of laughter. Offers laughter sessions, classes and workshops as well as a Telephone Laughter Club.
Email: info@laughternetwork.co.uk
Website: www.laughternetwork.co.uk

The London Sleep Centre

A private clinic that accepts referrals from GPs and direct patient referrals when patients are self-funding. It provides access to a range of services for those suffering from all types of sleep disorders. It also offers an online sleep assessment to help you determine whether you have a sleep disorder.
Telephone: 020 7725 0523
Website: www.londonsleepcentre.com

Medicines and Healthcare products Regulatory Agency (MHRA)

A government agency responsible for ensuring that medicines and medical devices work and are acceptably safe.
Address: 10–2 Market Towers, 1 Nine Elms Lane, London, SW8 5NQ
Telephone: 020 7084 2000 or020 7210 3000
Email: info@mhra.gsi.gov.uk
Website: www.mhra.gov.uk

Narcolepsy Association UK (UKAN)

A registered charity offering information and advice, including a newsletter, to sufferers of narcolepsy and their relatives. The charity also encourages research into the causes and treatment of the condition.
Address: PO Box 13842, Penicuik, EH26 8WX
Telephone: 0845 450 0394
Email: info@narcolepsy.org.uk
Website: www.narcolepsy.org.uk

National Sleep Foundation

An American independent non-profit organisation that aims to improve public health and safety by promoting understanding of sleep and sleep disorders and supporting sleep-related education, research and advocacy. The website offers a wide range of useful resources including online sleep assessment tools, quizzes and a forum.
Website: www.sleepfoundation.org.

Nytol The Good Sleep Guide

As well as providing product information, this website offers a wide range of information about sleep and an online version of the Epworth Sleepiness Scale to help you determine whether or not you get enough sleep.
Website: www.nytol.co.uk

Patient UK

Website that claims to offer the same information that a GP provides during a consultation. Gives a comprehensive overview of insomnia and provides articles on various aspects of the topic, as well as links to relevant news items and a patient experience forum. Also offers a printable sleep diary.
Website: www.patient.co.uk

Pillow Talk

The Mail on Sunday's weekly column about sleep, written by Dr Chris Idzikowski, director of the Edinburgh Sleep Centre. You can email your questions about sleep and sleep problems to Dr Idzikowski.
Email: pillowtalk@mailonsunday.co.uk

Relaxation for Living

Offers information on stress and its effects on the body as well as relaxation techniques. Also provides a database of Relaxation for Living Institute teachers and relaxation classes across the UK.
Address: Relaxation for Living, 1 Great Chapel Street, London, W1F 8FA
Telephone: 020 7439 4277 or 020 7437 5880
Website: www.rfli.co.uk

The Sleep Apnoea Trust Association

A leading UK Charity that works to help sufferers of sleep apnoea and their families.
Address: The Sleep Apnoea Trust,12a Bakers Piece, Kingston Blount, Oxon, OX39 4SW
Telephone: 0845 60 60 685
Website: www.sleep-apnoea-trust.org

The Sleep Council

A non-profit organisation funded by bed manufacturers, suppliers and retailers that offers advice on how to get a good night's sleep, including how to choose a new bed or mattress. The organisation also runs a helpline that offers support for insomnia sufferers.
Address: High Corn Mill, Chapel Hill, Skipton, North Yorkshire, BD23 1NL
Email: info@sleepcouncil.org.uk
Website: www.sleepcouncil.com

Sleep Education.com

A US website run by the American Academy of Sleep Medicine. Provides accurate information about sleep and sleep disorders plus the latest news on sleep medicine.

Website: www.sleepeducation.com

Sleep Matters

A nurse-run information line operated by the Medical Advisory Service.

Tel: 020 8994 9874

Website: www.medicaladvisoryservice.org.uk

Sleep Net

An American educational website devoted to improving sleep health worldwide.

Website: www.sleepnet.com

Sleep Research Centre, Loughborough University

One of the UK's leading sleep research centres. Offers general information about insomnia and other sleep disorders, including how to deal with sleep problems in babies and children. Also contains general articles about sleep by Professor Jim Horne.

Address: Sleep Research Centre, Loughborough University, Leicestershire, LE11 3TU

Telephone: 01509 223091

Email: Sleep.Research@lboro.ac.uk

Website: www.lboro.ac.uk/departments/hu/groups/sleep

Sleep Research Society

An American member organisation of scientists that aims to foster scientific investigation on all aspects of sleep and its disorders, to promote training and education in sleep research and to provide forums for the

exchange of knowledge pertaining to sleep. Publishes the journal Sleep in collaboration with the American Academy of Sleep Medicine.
Website: www.sleepresearchsociety.org

Talk About Sleep

An American website that aims to provide an online destination where patients, medical practitioners, healthcare professionals, academics, researchers and vendors can share ideas, concerns, experiences and enhance their knowledge of sleep-related issues. Membership is free and benefits include a free monthly newsletter and new product information.
Website: www.talkaboutsleep.com

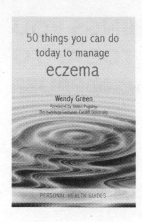

50 THINGS YOU CAN DO TODAY TO MANAGE ECZEMA

Wendy Green

ISBN: 978 84024 721 3

Paperback £4.99

Did you know that eczema affects one in five children and one in twelve adults in the UK?

Are you one of them?

In this easy-to-follow book, Wendy Green explains the psychological, dietary and hormonal factors that can cause eczema, and offers practical advice and a holistic approach to help you deal with the symptoms, including simple lifestyle and dietary changes and DIY complementary therapies.

'*This book provides a superb overview of eczema... The advice is up to date with current clinical research... offering the reader all they need to know to combine conventional and complementary treatments with a healthy lifestyle*'

Helen Pugsley, dermatology lecturer, Cardiff University

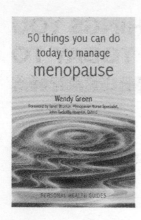

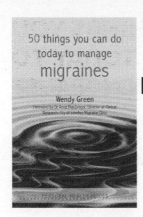

50 THINGS YOU CAN DO TODAY TO MANAGE MIGRAINES

Wendy Green

ISBN: 978 84024 722 0

Paperback £4.99

Do you suffer from severe headaches, sometimes with nausea and visual impairment?

Can these headaches last for up to a day or longer at a time?

If so, you could be experiencing migraines. In this easy-to-follow book, Wendy Green explains how dietary, psychological and environmental factors can cause migraines, and offers practical advice and a holistic approach to help you manage them, including simple lifestyle and dietary changes and DIY complementary therapies.

'Wendy Green outlines the variety of treatments that are available over the counter, and also gives an overview of what is available from a GP... It may not yet be possible to 'cure' migraines but it is possible to lead a normal life despite them'

Dr Anne MacGregor, director of clinical research,
City of London Migraine Clinic

www.summersdale.com

Have you enjoyed this book?
If so, why not write a review on your favourite website?
Thanks very much for buying this Summersdale book.